Human Tooth and Developmental Dental Defects - Compositional and Genetic Implications

Edited by Ana Gil de Bona and Hakan Karaaslan

Published in London, United Kingdom

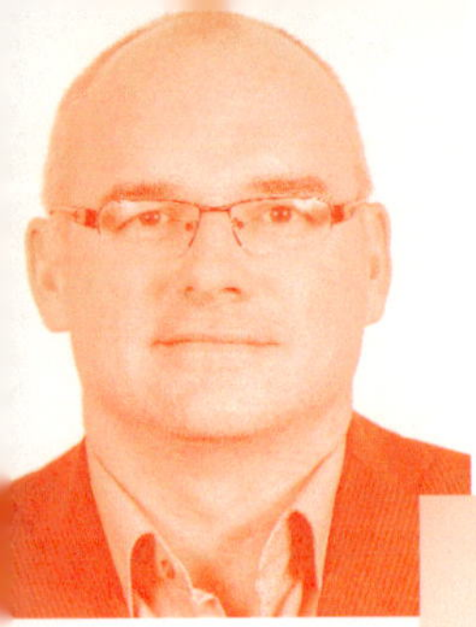
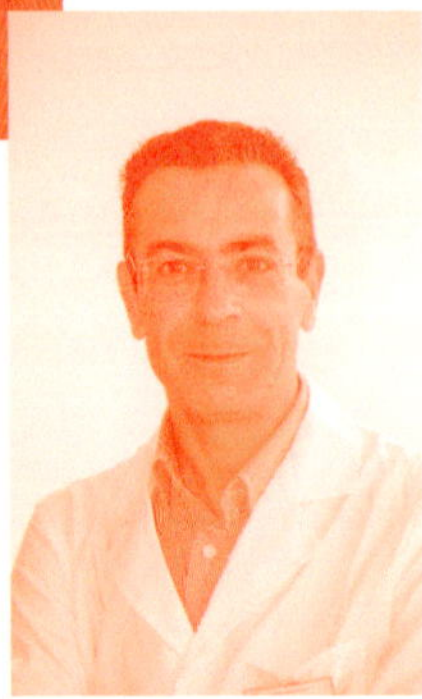
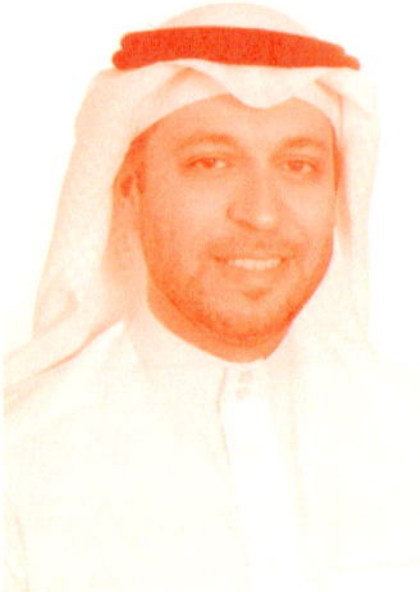
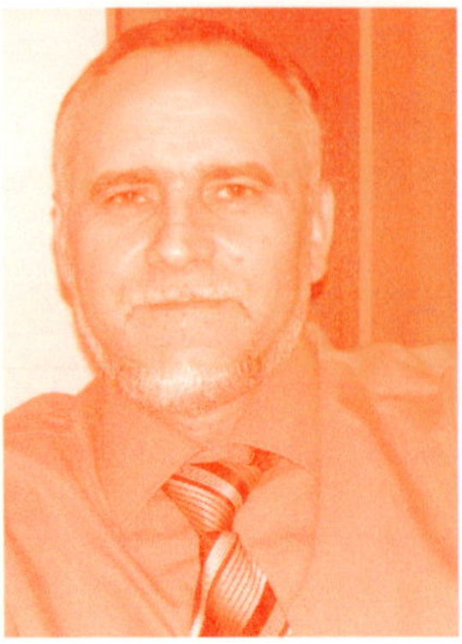
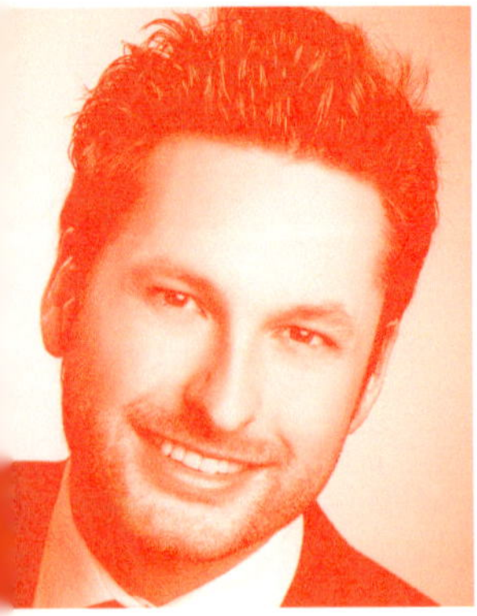
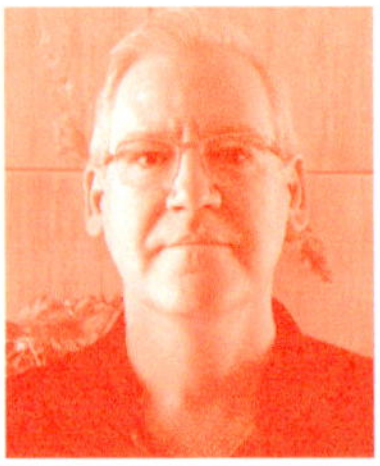
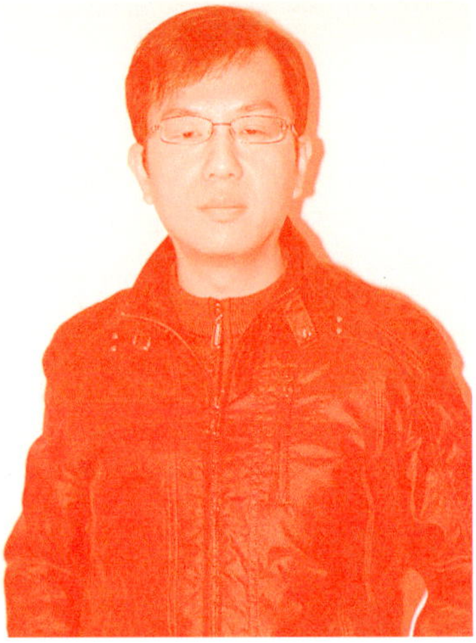

IntechOpen

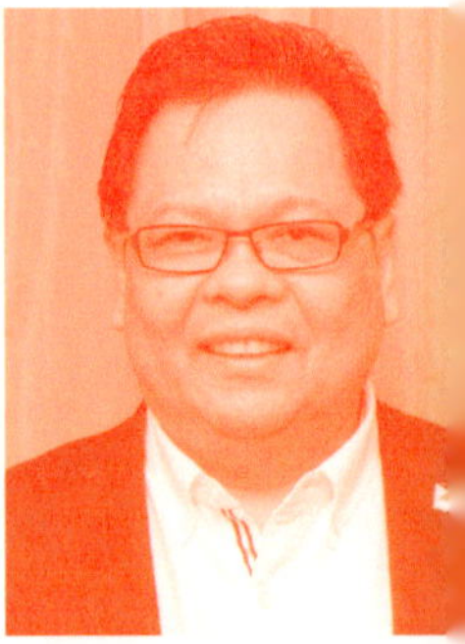
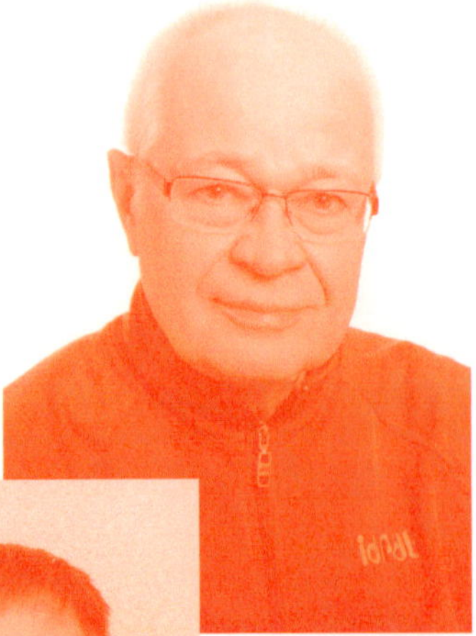
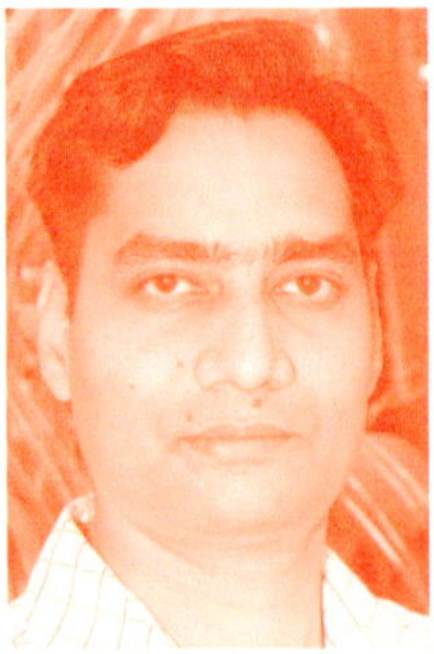
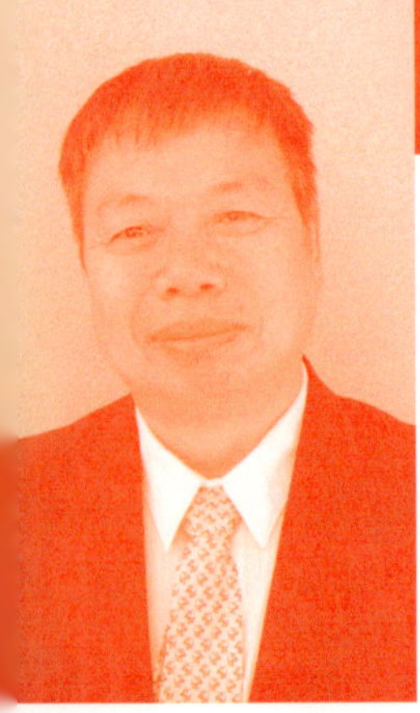
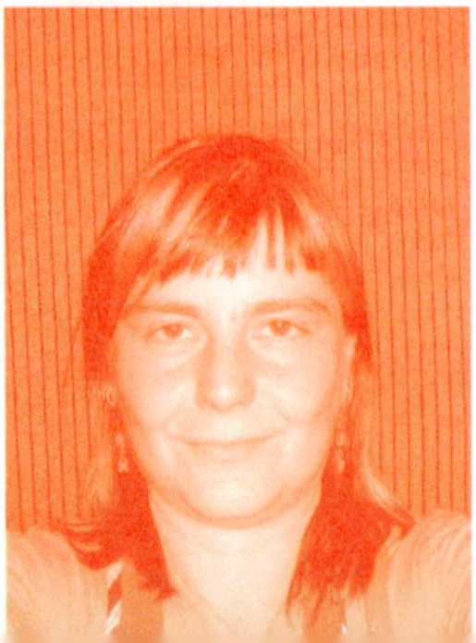
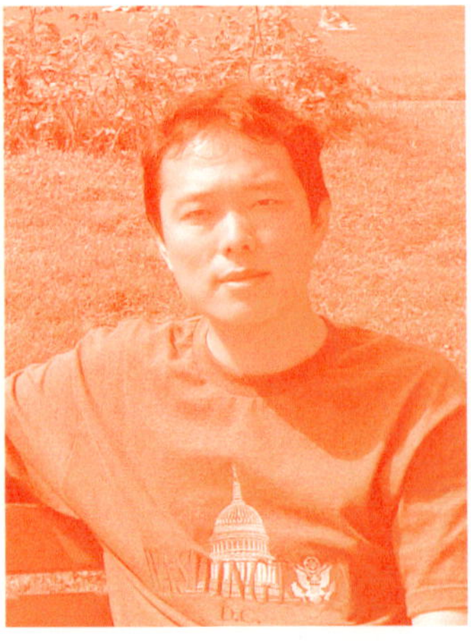

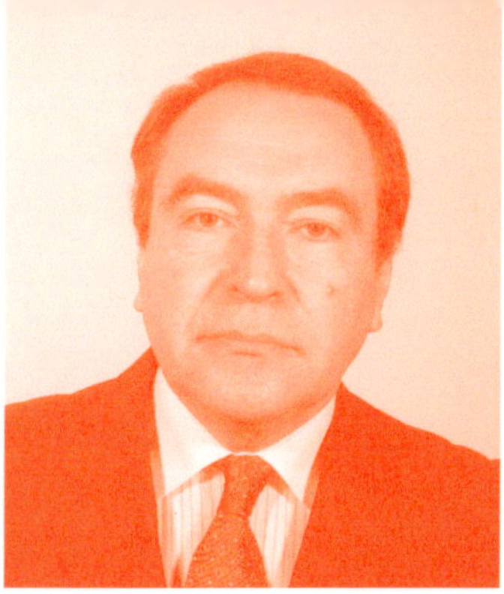
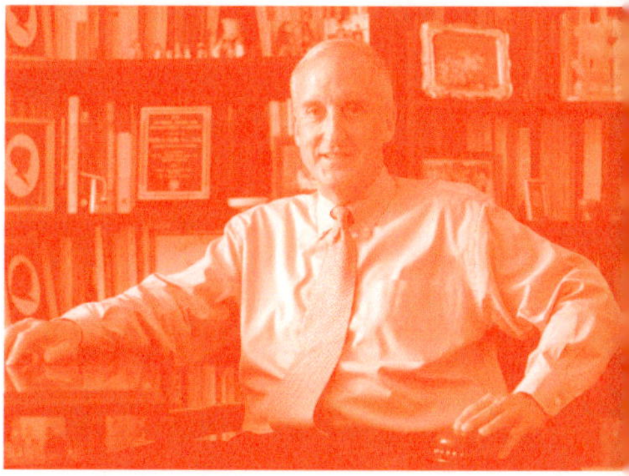
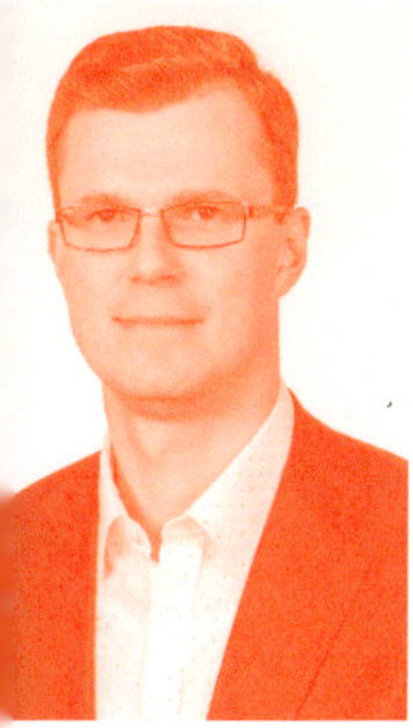
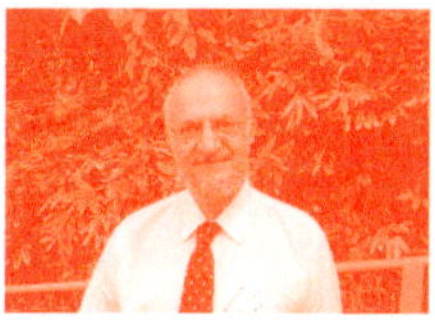
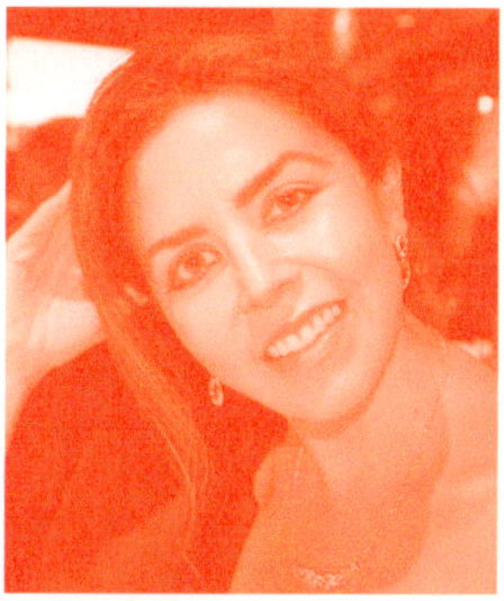

Supporting open minds since 2005

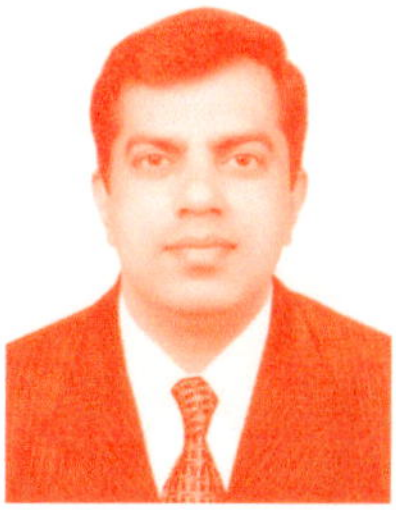
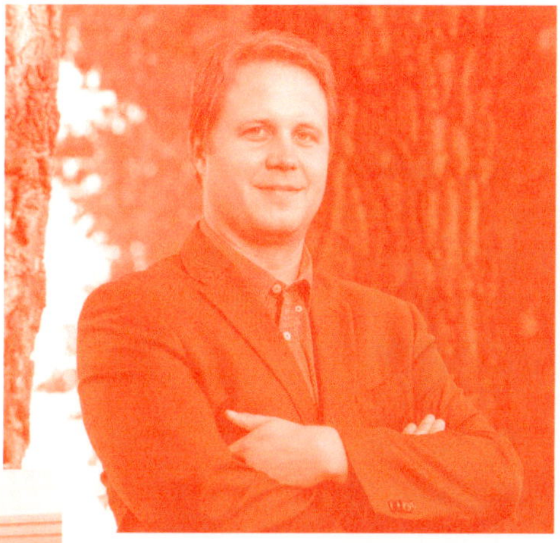
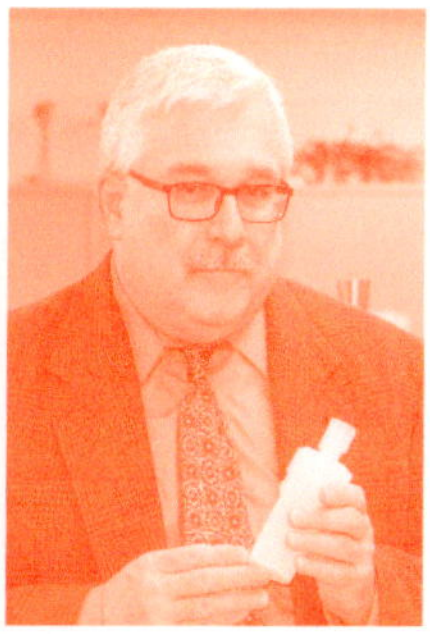
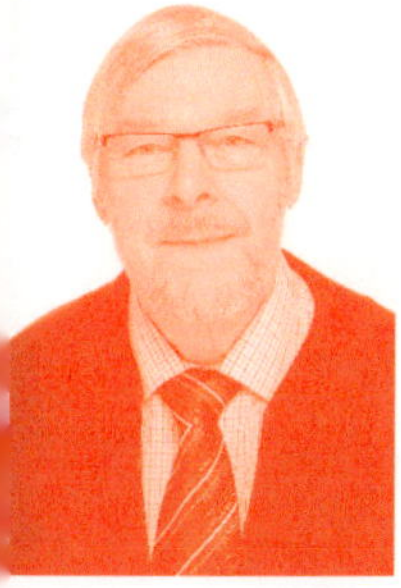
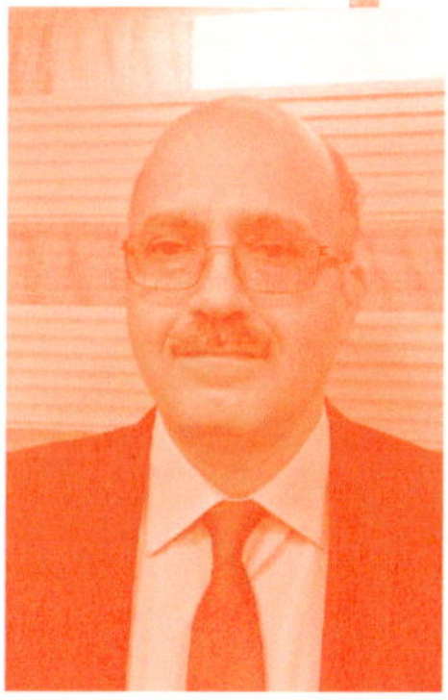
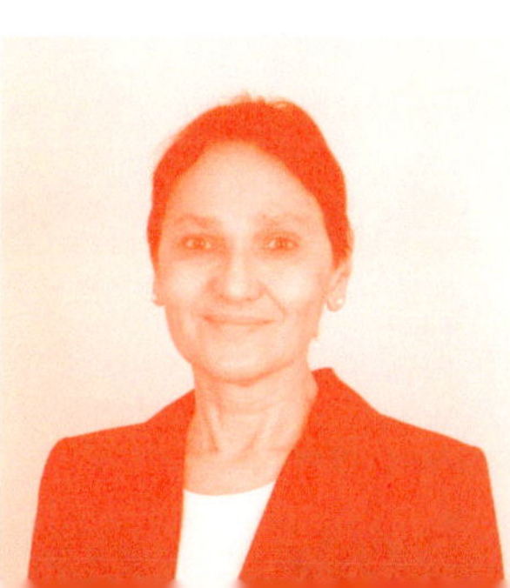
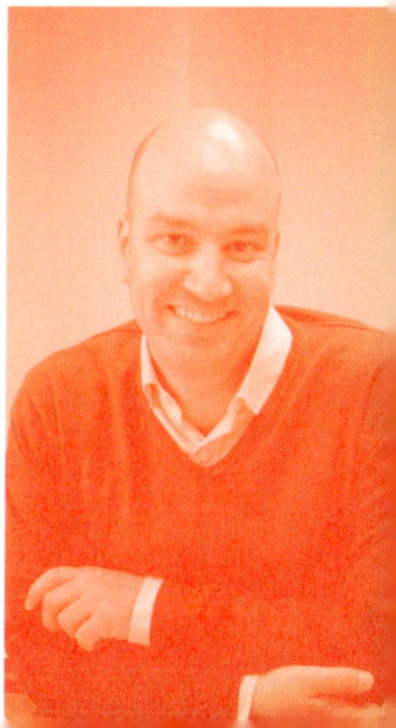

Human Tooth and Developmental Dental Defects - Compositional and Genetic Implications
http://dx.doi.org/10.5772/intechopen.92497
Edited by Ana Gil de Bona and Hakan Karaaslan

Contributors
Y.B. Yallappa Aswini, Kavita Rijhwani, Vikrant Mohanty, Emilia Severin, George Gabriel Moldoveanu, Andreea Moldoveanu, Antonio Liras, Luis Romeu, Luis Javier Serrano, Juan Andrés de Pablo, Mariano García-Arranz, Santo Catapano, Francesco Grande, Sukumar Athimoolam, In-Woong Um, Min-Keun Kim, Eui-Seok Lee, Puneet Wadhwa, Yu-Mi Kim, Heng Bo Jiang

First published in London, United Kingdom, 2022 by IntechOpen
IntechOpen is the global imprint of INTECHOPEN LIMITED, registered in England and Wales, registration number: 11086078, 5 Princes Gate Court, London, SW7 2QJ, United Kingdom
Printed in Croatia

British Library Cataloguing-in-Publication Data
A catalogue record for this book is available from the British Library

Additional hard and PDF copies can be obtained from orders@intechopen.com

Human Tooth and Developmental Dental Defects - Compositional and Genetic Implications
Edited by Ana Gil de Bona and Hakan Karaaslan
p. cm.
Print ISBN 978-1-83969-104-1
Online ISBN 978-1-83969-105-8
eBook (PDF) ISBN 978-1-83969-106-5

For EU product safety concerns:
IN TECH d.o.o., Prolaz Marije Krucifikse Kozulić 3, 51000 Rijeka, Croatia, info@intechopen.com or visit our website at intechopen.com.

Meet the editors

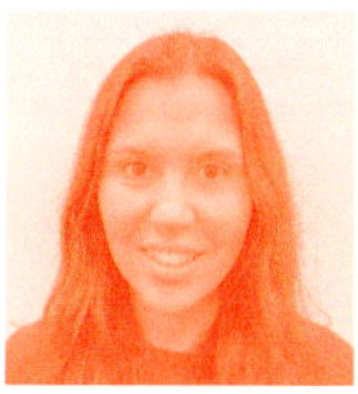

Dr. Ana Gil de Bona received her Ph.D. in Molecular Biology and Microbiology from Complutense University of Madrid, Spain. Her research mainly focused on the study of the proteomic profile of the extracellular vesicles and the secretome in virulent and avirulent strains of Candida albicans. She continued her scientific career at the University of Massachusetts Medical School, USA, working in yeast genetics and proteomics. Her current research at the Forsyth Institute, USA, is focused on understanding the changes in tooth enamel in healthy and defective teeth to find better diagnostics tools and treatment approaches. She has authored peer-reviewed research articles and reviews and has presented her work at national and international scientific meetings.

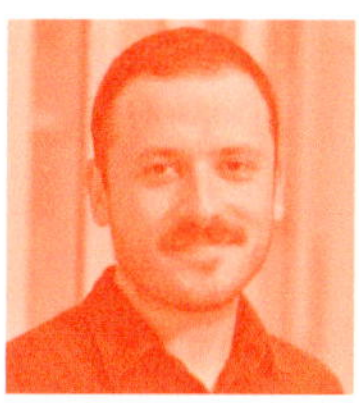

Dr. Hakan Karaaslan completed his endodontic training at Hacettepe University, Turkey, where he received his DDS. His post-graduate thesis work focused on the mineral content and structure of dentin exposed to bleaching agents. Pursuing his interest in understanding the development and structure of dental hard tissues, he worked at Dr. Tim Bromage's Lab at New York University on the incremental nature of enamel. At the Forsyth Institute, USA, Dr. Karaaslan currently investigates developmental dental defects, in particular molar hypomineralization, furthering his passion for hard tissue biology. As an endodontist and a clinician, he also seeks to understand the pulpal aspect of enamel defects and translate basic science findings into clinical therapeutics.

Contents

Preface

Covered by dental enamel, supported by dentin and cementum, and given life by the pulp in its core, the human tooth is indeed an extraordinary tissue. Despite this, teeth are often affected by dental caries or cavities. Research on dental hard tissues and their developmental pathologies is attracting more attention from the scientific community. This book presents the basics of developmental dental defects, which affect a large population worldwide and thus require new preventive and therapeutical approaches.

This book is organized into two sections. Section 1, "The Components of Dental Hard Tissues and Developmental Dental Defects," covers the basics of the human tooth while emphasizing the importance of organic content and trace elements. These components are responsible for giving the unique chemical and mechanical properties of dental hard tissues along with the hydroxyapatite-based mineral phase.

Section 2, "Genetic Components of Developmental Dental Defects," elucidates the complex genetic machinery behind tooth development. It provides an introduction to the genetic and epigenetic basis of developmental dental defects and directs the reader to the relevant literature.

This book presents the basics of developmental dental defects in chapters written by experts from all over the world. We are confident that students, scientists, and clinicians from diverse backgrounds will find this book useful and we hope the information contained herein contributes to future research in the field.

Ana Gil de Bona and Hakan Karaaslan
The Forsyth Institute,
Harvard School of Dental Medicine,
Cambridge, Massachusetts, USA

Section 1

The Components of Dental Hard Tissues and Developmental Dental Defects

Chapter 1

Organic Matrix of Enamel and Dentin and Developmental Defects

Eui-Seok Lee, Puneet Wadhwa, Min-Keun Kim, Heng Bo Jiang, In-Woong Um and Yu-Mi Kim

Abstract

The anatomical crown of the tooth is covered by enamel and root is covered by cementum. The dentin forms the major part of the tooth. The dentin structure is very similar to that of the bone both physically and chemically which is why many scientists have wondered about using its properties for developing a novel bone graft material. In contrast with hard and brittle enamel dentin is viscoelastic. The organic structure of dentin which is about 35% is composed of mainly type *I* collagen embedded in mucopolysaccharides ground substance. Approximately half of the non-collagenous composition consists of hyperphosphorylated proteins. The acidic glycoproteins, Gla-proteins, serum proteins, proteoglycans etc. composes the remaining part. The dentin matrix consists of many similar proteins as that of bone like dentin phosphoprotein, dentin sialoprotein etc.. The matrix also consists of many growth factors. Any external disturbance like an infection, trauma, calcium or phosphorous metabolic changes can lead to defective amelogenesis. Mutational changes can lead to defect in dentin. An early diagnosis can result in a satisfactory treatment plan contributing to functional and esthetical compensation.

Keywords: Enamel matrix, Dentin matrix, Tooth proteins, Growth factors, Tooth developmental defects

1. Introduction

Enamel and dentin constitute different concentrations of organic, water and mineral contents. This accounts for their specific physical-mechanical properties and their integration allow the tooth to be functionally stable in adverse oral conditions [1]. Dentin tissue underlines the enamel and constitutes the bulk of the tooth. The inorganic to organic ratio is different in various tissues, these variations affect the properties of these tissues. The enamel is tougher and most highly resistant to force in comparison to other hard tissue in the body owing to its high inorganic content. On the other hand the dentin with high organic content serves as a resilient layer under enamel and cementum [2]. Enamel shows higher mineralization than cementum as there is more carbon 49% (wt) in cementum than enamel 3% (wt). Enamel being the hardest tissue and dentin being softer whereas X-ray diffraction (XRD) shows cementum has poorest crystallinity. Following decalcification process for separation of organic and inorganic content the organic components of the dentin are retained thereby maintaining the dentin shape. However due to 90% mineral content of the enamel it is lost after decalcification.

2. Enamel

Tooth enamel possess remarkable structural and mechanical properties making it an unique tissue. Tooth enamel is a complex mineralized tissue comprising of long and parallel apatite crystals configured into decussating enamel rods [3, 4]. The enamel consists of 96% inorganic and 4% organic and water content and is the most mineralized tissue. The organic content of enamel is less than that of dentin. The organic content consist of some unique proteins present only in enamel and lipids [5]. The enamel is formed only once before the eruption of the tooth. Following eruption the tooth organ permanently loses the ability to form new enamel [3].

Being highly mineralized enamel could be expected to be brittle and have low fracture resistance. However, the experimental studies proved that the fracture toughness of enamel is equivalent to or even better than some tough ceramics [6, 7].

2.1 Enamel proteins

During the development of enamel, ameloblasts secrete enamel matrix protein. Proteins are large complex molecules that are required for the structure, function and regulating body's tissues and organs. Enamel matrix proteins bind to the hydroxyapatite structuring the enamel and modulating crystal growth [8, 9]. Initial developing enamel matrix constitutes 60-70% water, 20-30% proteins and 15-20% of mineral ions. Mineralization process leads to resorption of enamel proteins and water leaving very little amount of organic content in matured enamel [3]. Major components of the enamel matrix protein (EMP) are the amelogenins constituting greater than 90% of all the organic content in the enamel [10, 11]. The other type of protein group is the non – amelogenin including enamelins, tuftelin and sheathlins. Other than these two enzymes, matrix metalloproteinase (MMP)-20 and enamel matrix serine proteinase (EMSP)-1 are also present in the EMP (**Figure 1**) [10].

Enamel proteins consist of 1-2% of the total composition. These proteins are located mainly at the enamel rods interface. The proteins play a role in modulation of the stress in enamel and contributes to the elastic and viscoelastic behavior [12]. Any kind of damage or denaturation of the enamel or dentin non-collagenous proteins can decrease the durability of the tooth [12]. Tooth whitening procedures or treatment with potassium hydroxide leads to loss of enamel proteins causing enamel to be more prone to fracture [12, 13]. Radiation therapy for treatment of oral cancers is also known to damage the enamel proteins [12]. In a study the enamel proteins were extracted using potassium hydroxide treatment from the

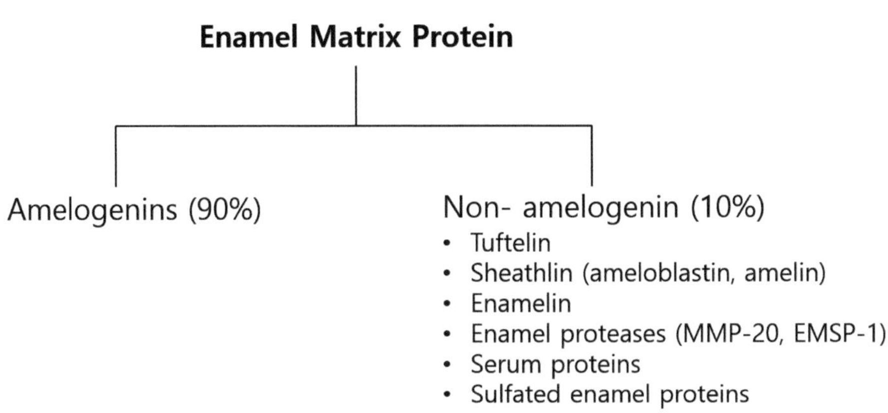

Figure 1.
Types of enamel matrix proteins.

enamel sections of the molar cusps. The results showed a 40% reduction in fracture toughness in comparison with a fully proteinized control. The organic content of the enamel is very small, but it is of importance crack growth toughening. This is because it helps in forming unbroken ligament and fortify its efficacy [14].

The synthesis and secretion of the organic extracellular matrix is controlled by ameloblasts and deposited along the dentino-enamel junction which eventually controls enamel biomineralization [15].

Amelogenins are hydrophobic in nature, they are rich in proline (25%), glutamine (14%), leucine (9%) and histidine (7%) amino acid residues [4, 15]. Amelogenin functions in regulating orientation, shape and length of enamel crystals [16]. Tuftelin is suggested to function at the level of ameloblast differentiation, it may play a role in extracellular matrix secretion. Tuftelin is also expressed in different soft tissues, which suggest it may have multifunctional role [17]. Ameloblastin also known as sheathlin and amelin present in Tomes' processes of the secretory ameloblasts the sheath space between rod and inter-rod enamel suggest that this protein may play a role in biomineralization. Enamelin is also believed to play a role in enamel

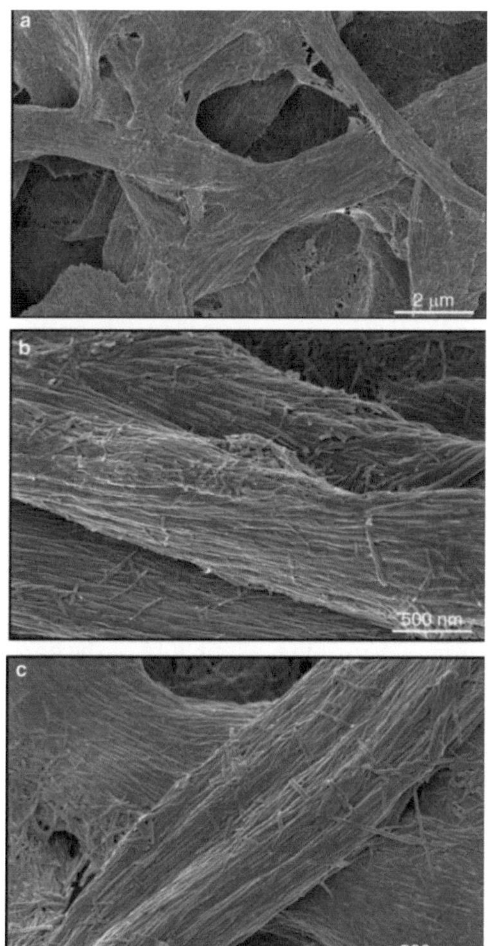

Figure 2.
Scanning electron micrograph images of engineered enamel. In this study apatite was grown within a decellularized enamel protein matrix, resulting in decussating enamel prisms containing distinct and separated individual enamel crystals. A SEM image overview of the engineered enamel apatite, b depicts parallel bundles of enamel crystals, and c depicts newly formed decussating enamel rods [3]. Figure adapted from Pandya M et al. (2019).

biomineralization. Enamelin is hydrophilic and an acidic protein rich in glycine, aspartic acid and serine [4]. The enamel proteins with unique properties requires specific proteases for their removal during enamel maturation whose spatiotemporal expression is impeccably regulated. This requirement is met by serine protease kallikrein-4 and MMP20 [18]. Enamel proteases processes secreted amelogenins, ameloblastin and enamelin in the matrix and eventually degrades and remove them from the mineralizing matrix when maturation of amelogenesis occurs. The sulfated enamel proteins are present in very small amount in the enamel matrix [15].

2.2 Applications of enamel matrix proteins

Enamel matrix derivative (EMD) is approved by FDA to be used as a material for periodontal regeneration since 1997 [19]. EMD is commercially obtained by heat treated lyophilized proteins that are isolated from porcine enamel at specific stage of development [20]. Emdogain, a mixture of enamel matrix proteins mainly composed of amelogenin is used for repair of hard and soft periodontal tissues [11, 21–23]. Emdogain has shown similar results to guided tissue regeneration with added advantage of easy to use with minimal complications [23].

Owing to its unique properties like toughness and relative fracture resistance researchers are focusing on developing an enamel-like biomaterial. Enamel biomimetics hold a great promise as structural components in a wide range of fields for biomedical and engineering applications. Some examples are like tooth repair, restoring a orthopedic defect site, functional insulator components, brakes and exhaust pollutant filters [3, 24]. Enamel proteins and calcium phosphate growth solutions seems to be a convincing formulation for biologically synthesizing tooth enamel. Based on the established role of enamel proteins, using an EMP researchers were successfully grew elongated and parallel apatite crystals within decussating enamel prisms (**Figure 2**) [3]. The research until now using biochemical approaches can only mimic limited features of apatite and calcium phosphate crystal growth.

3. Dentin

The dentin consists of 65% inorganic and 35% organic and water content. The presence of more organic content in dentin than enamel makes it very similar to that of bone. The organic part of dentin is composed of collagenous fibrils embedded in ground substance of mucopolysacchrides [5]. Type I collagen is the principal type of collagen in dentin. It contributes about 90% of the organic content, the remaining 10% contains several proteins and proteoglycans, acidic glycoproteins referred to as non-collagenous proteins [25, 26]. Also type I collagen is abundantly present organic constituent of the bone extracellular matrix [27]. The collagen fibrils form a scaffold network and are densely mineralized. The dentin consists of little amounts of type V and III collagen. The odontoblasts synthesize and secretes the non-collagenous proteins as well collagen fibrils [28].

Dentin constitutes tubules ranging in size of micrometer and surrounded by highly mineralized peritubular dentin, embedded in a matrix rich in collagen called intertubular dentin. Lamina limitans a sheet-like structure divide the peritubular and the intertubular dentin and primarily composed of proteoglycans protein cores. The proteoglycans contribute to mechanical behavior of dentin. They link the collagen fibrils securing the collagenous network together [12]. Peritubular dentin is primarily made of glycosaminoglycans and lacks collagen fibrils [29]. Intertubular matrix chiefly constitutes type I collagen fibrils with non-collagenous proteins and proteoglycans which forms a three-dimensional organic network buttressed by apatite mineral crystallites [30].

The adhesive systems used for dentin bonding rely on formation of a hybrid layer. This hybrid layer is formed by demineralized collagen fibrils reinforced by resin matrix. As the resin monomers are unable to infiltrate the mineralized tissues, so adhesive bonding systems are used which has an acid, primer and an adhesive. The acid helps in removing mineral crystals and exposing the collagen. The primer which is a hydrophilic solution permits the infiltration of resin monomer into the demineralized dentin. Finally, the adhesive consisting of a mixture of monomers penetrates the treated surface thereby forming mechanical adhesion with dentin. Removing the unbound water from hybrid layer and suppressing the endogenous enzymatic activity have helped in increasing biocompatibility by inhibiting degradation of the hybrid layer [31].

3.1 Dentin proteins

The dentin matrix and bone proteins are similar. Type I collagen designs an effective and instructional template for guiding deposition of calcium phosphate polymorphs and subsequently transforming into crystalline hydroxyapatite crystals. The highly complex process of hydroxyapatite nucleation and collagen mineralization is also controlled by non-collagenous proteins. The amount of these non-collagenous proteins in dentin and bone is small, but they play an indispensable role in bone formation and remodeling. Some examples of non-collagenous proteins found in both are osteocalcin, osteopontin and bone sialoprotein. The dentin matrix proteins are of interest because of their calcium binding property in the extracellular matrix which leads to calcification of tissue [32]. Many studies have shown similarities between dentin and bone. Apart from type I collagen being the leading extracellular matrix element, other common proteins and proteoglycans are osteonectin/SPARC, osteocalcin, osteopontin, bone sialoprotein, decorin and biglycan [33].

Dentin proteoglycans plays a key role in mineralization of the dentin and bone, so they perform structural, metabolic, and functional role. The proteoglycans are classified as small leucine-rich proteoglycans (SLRP) and the large aggregating proteoglycans. The SLRP are further divided into 5 classes: decorin; biglycan; fibromodulin; lumican and osteoadherin. Among the large aggregating proteoglycan is only versican has been described well in dentin [25].

Osteocalcin and osteonectin are classified under secretory calcium-binding phosphoprotein a category of non-collagenous proteins. Osteocalcin is a vitamin K-dependent gamma-carboxylated protein. It is a small calcium binding protein consisting of three glutamic acid residues. It is found in dentin in small amounts as compared to the bone [25]. Osteonectin binds collagen, hydroxyapatite and growth factors. It is known to regulate proliferation of cells, prompts angiogenesis and formulation of matrix metalloproteinases [34]. Another subset of the secretory calcium binding phosphoprotein is the Small Integrin-Binding ligand, N-linked Glycoprotein (SIBLING) family. It includes osteopontin, bone sialoprotein, dentin matrix protein 1, dentin sialophosphoprotein, and matrix extracellular phosphoglycoprotein [35].

Dentin phosphoprotein (DPP) and dentin sialoprotein (DSP) were earlier thought to be unique to dentin [5, 33]. Later some immunohistochemical studies established that DSP is also present in the alveolar bone, cellular cementum, osteocytes, cementocytes and their matrices [36]. DPP is rich in aspartic acid and phosphoserine and bind calcium in considerable amounts. DSP is a glycoprotein rich in aspartic acid, serine, glutamic acid, and glycine. Both DPP and DSP are synthesized by odontoblasts and pre-ameloblast cell types. In contrast the bone matrix proteins are not exclusively made by the osteoblasts. This makes dentin unusual based on these dentin specific proteins [33]. DSP has been shown to play a role in prompting differentiation of dental pulp cells in odontoblast-like cells [36].

3.2 Dentin growth factors

Growth factors are natural activation signals or substances able to stimulate cellular proliferation, wound healing, and sometimes cellular differentiation. Generally, a growth factor is secreted protein or a steroid hormone [37, 38]. They are necessary for regulating various cellular processes that take part in tissue regeneration procedure [39, 40].

Growth factors are generally acting as signaling molecules between the cells, like cytokines and hormones binding to specific receptors on the target cells surfaces. Examples of growth factors in dentin are TGF- β group, BMP group, Insulin growth factor-1, hepatocyte growth factor, VEGF, Adrenomedullin, FGF-2, platelet-derived growth factor, growth/differentiation factor etc. a summary of these growth factors is given in **Table 1**.

We can group these growth factors by their actions as: Angiogenisis (FGF-2, PDGF, VEGF, NGF); Differentiation (TGF-β, PDGF, FGF-2, BMPs, IGF, NGF); Proliferation (PDGF, FGF-2, IGF, VEGF, TGF-β, SDF-1); Chemotaxis (PDGF, FGF-2, TGF-β, SDF-1) and Neuronal growth (NGF) [41].

Transforming growth factor-beta	
TGF-β1	Promoting tertiary dentinogenesis and in primary odontoblastic differentiation.
TGF-β2	Upregulated on DPSCs differentiation into a mineralizing phenotype
TGF-β3	Promotes odontoblastic differentiation
Bone morphogenetic proteins	
BMP-2	Promotes vitro and in vivo odontoblastic differentiation, DSPP induction and increases alkaline phosphatase activity
BMP-4	Increases odontoblastic differentiation
BMP-7	Promotes DPSCs phenotype mineralization
Insulin growth factor-1	Promotes proliferation and differentiation of DPSCs and SCAP into a mineralizing phenotype
fibroblast growth factor 2 (FGF-2)	Promotes stem cell homing (chemotaxis), angiogenesis, and stemness
Platelet-derived growth factor	Promotes angiogenesis, chemotaxis of MSCs modulates the process of odontoblastic differentiation, synergistic act with other growth factors
Growth/differentiation factor 15	Promotes axonal function and regeneration after injury and plays important role in neuronal maintenance
Vascular endothelial growth factor VEGF	Potent angiogenic factor that promotes blood vessel formation in tooth slices implanted subcutaneously in SCID mice
Hepatocyte growth factor	Promotes survival, proliferation, and migration of MSCs
Adrenomedullin	Promotes odontoblastic differentiation through activation of p38
Epidermal growth factor	Enhances neurogenic differentiation of DPSCs and SCAP
Placenta growth factor	Promotes osteogenic and angiogenesis differentiation of MSCs
Brain-derived neurotrophic factor	Promotes neuronal growth and axonal targeting
Glial cell line-derived neurotrophic factor	Promotes in vivo nerve regeneration and pulp cell proliferation. Increased expression during odontogenic differentiation.

Table 1.
Growth factors in dentin matrix and their role.

The growth factors diffusion into the dentinal-pulpal junction is postulated to activate reactionary dentinogenesis and simultaneous reparative dentinogenesis along with pulp tissue inflammatory reaction [42, 43]. The surviving odontoblasts secrete reactionary dentin as a response to environmental stimuli causing metabolic activity increase in the cells. The inductive molecules determining the success of the pulp healing might be released from damaged dentin and adjacent pulp tissue [44]. Dentin-pulp regeneration process can vary as it depends on the causative agent whether trauma or pathological conditions. An inflammatory reaction is caused by these events, which is supposed to be the beginning of tissue regeneration process [39]. Dentin-pulp defensive and reparative mechanisms mimic the embryonic tooth development stage and growth factors derived from dentin may play a key role in regulating these events [42]. The dentinal matrix constitutes angiogenic growth factors and their release after injury can contribute to overall reparative response of the dentinal-pulpal complex [45].

There are multiple growth factors in dentin that also exist in bone like insulin-like growth factor-1 (IGF-1), insulin-like growth factor-2 (IGF-2), transforming growth factor-beta (TGF-β), fibroblast growth factors (FGFs), platelet-derived growth factor (PDGF), parathyroid bone morphogenetic proteins (BMPs), and certain members of the growth differentiation factor (GDF) group of proteins [46–48]. That is why recent studies have shown good results after using dentin as a bone graft and stated that dentin has shown to be clinically safe and has good bone-forming capacity [49, 50].

Also known as autogenous tooth biomaterial it is derived from an extracted tooth through demineralization process. It is useful as graft material because of its osteoconductive properties [51]. This biomaterial can be used alone or combined with other materials for example with platelet-rich fibrin [52], bone marrow mesenchymal stem cells [53] or bone morphogenetic protein (BMP-2) [54] for enhanced bone regeneration effects. Recently a dentin derived barrier membrane acting as an osteoinductive collagen membrane showed successful outcome in guided bone regeneration and dental implantation. The membrane was derived from block type autogenous demineralized dentin matrix with advantage of overcoming the mechanical instability of the collagen membrane. It is mostly composed of type I collagen, making it suitable for use in implant procedures [55].

4. Dental defects

Enamel has 3 essential enamel proteins to build healthy well mineralized enamel which is secreted from ameloblasts "amelogenin, ameloblastin and enamelin" with the help of two enzymes, MMP20 and kallikrein-4 (Klk4) to form the enamel properly and sequent proteolysis of enamel protein [56]. In the event of alteration in the process of protein removal, enamel and dental defects will emerge like for example, amelogenesis imperfecta (AI), Chalky/Molar Hypomolarization (MH), Dentinogenesis Imperfecta (DI) or fluorosis [57]. **Figure 3** depicts the protein content in healthy and diseased tooth.

4.1 Amelogenesis imperfecta (AI)

Amelogenesis imperfecta is a rare, inherited enamel development disorder where mutations in the amelogenin gene results in malformation of the enamel layer. It is subdivided to 4 main types hypoplastic (type I), hypomaturation (type II), hypocalcified (type III), hypomaturation/hypoplasia/taurodontism (type IV).

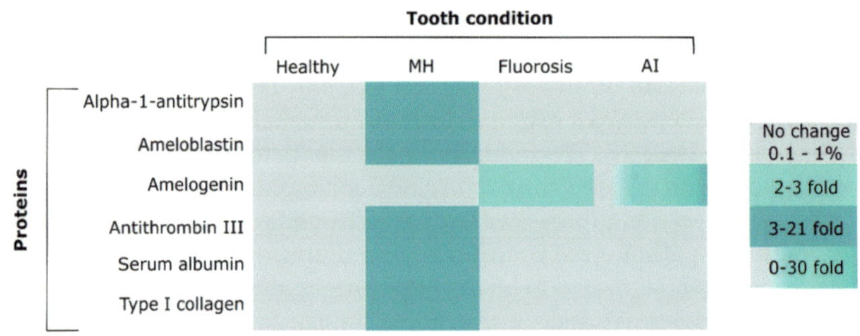

Figure 3.
Protein content is compared between healthy and diseased tooth enamel. Different proteins are presented in (rows) as analyzed different tooth conditions (columns). Healthy teeth is presented as reference in light gray, chalky/molar Hypomolarization (MH): Enamel affected by molar hypomineralization, fluorosis and Amelogenesis imperfecta (AI): Hypocalcified and hypomaturation amelogenesis imperfecta enamel; range of percent by weight (wt %) of protein abundance in comparison to healthy enamel show in 4 colors: Healthy range of 0.1–1 wt % (light gray); 2–3 times increase (light teal); 3–30 times increase (dark teal); 0–30 times increase (gray-teal gradient) [57]. Figure adapted from Gil-Bona a et al. (2020).

Clinical and radiographical features and enamel thickness, of different subtypes are dependent on mode of inheritance and gene mutation. AI occurs due to mutations in several genes, including enamelin, amelogenin, MMP20, Klk4 and FAM83H [58–61]. The mutations can lead to hypoplastic, hypomature, or hypocalcified form of the enamel [62]. AI can be easily seen clinically and radiographically as teeth appears in abnormal color like (yellow, brown, or gray). Soft enamel, due to hypo calcification enamel surface are more susceptible to caries, tooth attrition, teeth hypersensitivity, calculus formation, and gingivitis/periodontitis [63].

Type I hypoplastic AI has reduced thickness of enamel and shows pitting and grooves. In radiographs enamel shows normal contrasts from dentine. Type II hypomaturation AI has enamel of normal thickness but appearance is mottled. It is less severe than hypocalcified type. Radiographically it exhibits similar radiodensity as dentine. Type III hypocalcified AI have defect in enamel calcification. The enamel thickness is normal but is weak in structure and appearance is opaque and chalky. In radiographs enamel is less radio-opaque in comparison to dentin. Type IV hypomaturation/hypoplasia/taurodontism AI exhibits mixed hypomaturation and hypoplasia appearance. In taurodontism enlargement of the body and pulp chamber is observed. The pulp chamber floor and furcation moves apically down the root [58].

A proper diagnosis identifying the different phenotypes is essential to determine molecular etiology. The treatment plan aims at early diagnosis, managing the pain and restoring the defects with regular follow ups [58]. Mild variations can be treated adequately with facial veneers, whereas in severe cases full coverage is mandatory. For young patients milled acetal resin overlays can be used until fully erupted [64].

4.2 Chalky/molar hypomineralrisation (MH)

It is discolored white patches in one or more molars, porous dental enamel leads to hypersensitivity and risk of caries. Chalky enamel opacities contained unusually high amounts of protein, including serum albumin and other derivatives of blood and saliva [65]. Moderate and severe cases with opacities having a chalky texture exhibit failure of enamel surface soon after the eruption of tooth, it provides a hygiene-resistant nidus for dental plaque accumulation. The porous chalky enamel is invaded by accelerated decay which arises the need for restoration, extraction, or orthodontic treatment. It is observed that MH affects the 2-year molars or 6-year molars, a better understanding of its etiology is necessary [66]. Earlier systemic disturbance of enamel-forming cells (ameloblasts) during the hardening (maturation) stage of enamel formation was thought to be the cause [67]. A different pathomechanism indicating localized exposure of enamel to serum albumin was recently identified [68]. In a recent study the dose–response relationship between albumin and the enamel chalkiness was established. This supports the new pathomechanism also termed as "mineralization poisoning" [66].

MH is a complex problem requiring combinational treatment modalities. The treatment aim may be preventive or symptom control. Various treatment modalities can be adhesive and sealant restoration, composite restoration, glass ionomer restoration, preformed metal crown, microabrasion, bleach or orthodontic extraction [69].

4.3 Fluorosis

Dental fluorosis is a very common developmental disturbance that is caused by repeated exposures to high concentrations of fluoride during tooth or enamel formation. This leads to disturbance in enamel formation as the fluoride decreases calcium concentration in the matrix. This interferes with protease activity and delays or inhibit enamel matrix protein degradation. An abnormal apatite crystals growth occurs which leads to physical tooth surface changes [70]. It differs from white striations to stained pitting of the enamel depending on case severity [71]. The use of topical fluoride dentifrices in young children may increase the risk of dental fluorosis. In case of concern for fluorosis, in children under 6 years of age toothpaste with fluoride concentration less than 1000 parts per million should be used [70].

Treatment of the case depends on the severity and the esthetics concerns. Mild cases can be treated by bleaching if the tooth. For moderate cases enamel microabrasion with acids can be done. Composite fillings, veneers and crowns can be used for treating cases with severe forms of the disease [72].

The best solution for this condition is to control the fluoride intake for prevention of dental fluorosis [71].

4.4 Dentinogenesis imperfecta (DI)

DI is also an inherited condition also called "dentin dysplasia" with discolored teeth but most often blue-gray or yellow-brown which leads to wear, breakage, and loss of teeth. This damage can include teeth fractures or small holes (pitting) in the enamel. The enamel may have hypoplastic or hypocalcified defect in nearly one-third of patients and has tendency to crack away from defective dentin. It is a localized mesodermal dysplasia which affects both primary and permanent dentition. It is inherited in simple autosomal dominant mode exhibiting high penetrance and low mutation rate [73].

DI has 3 types: Type I: occurs in people who have osteogenesis imperfecta so, it appears to have other health concern (mutation in COL1A1/A2 gene). Type II: the most common type occurs in people without another inherited disorder (mutation in DSPP). Radiographically it shows complete obliteration of the pulp cavity by dentin. Type II and type III, are actually similar conditions but in different forms but DI type III shows enlarged pulp cavities [63].

In histological findings although enamel is normal in structure it tends to crack. Scalloping is absent in dentino-enamel junction. Mostly mantle dentin structure is normal. However dentinal tubules of the circumferential dentin are found to be coarse and branched. The tubules are reduced in quantity. An atubular area is present in the dentin with reduction in mineralization and decreased number of odontoblasts. Another common finding is pulpal inclusions and much interglobular dentin [73].

Treatment differs from case to case depend on its severity and presenting pain, also the patient age. Mostly treatments are targeted at maintaining oral hygiene and esthetics. Early diagnosis and treatment can prevent deterioration of teeth and occlusion. In severe cases two treatment stages for primary teeth under general anesthesia is recommended. At the age of 18-20 months the stage 1 treatment involves composite restorations covering for incisors and preformed crowns for first primary molars. At the age of 28-30 months stage 2 aims at protecting second primary molars and canines. For moderate cases one-stage treatment for primary teeth at 30 months of age is optimal. In severe cases composite restoration may not be helpful. A long term follow-up is necessary to adjust treatment according to change in dentition and occlusion [73].

5. Conclusion

The enamel and dentin organic content varies in amount and its constituents. The enamel proteins help in imparting the elastic and visco-elastic properties to the enamel. The clinical significance of the non-collagenous proteins may be in relation with dentinal growth factor release by calcium hydroxide or mineral trioxide aggregate. The dentin organic matrix constitutes similarity with that of bone, makes it a desirable bone graft material. Demineralized dentin autogenous bone grafts have already been used for dental implant surgeries and provides an easy to prepare and use bone graft material. Any imbalance in the organic content can manifest as developmental disease of the tooth.

Conflict of interest

The authors declare no conflict of interest.

Author details

Eui-Seok Lee[1†], Puneet Wadhwa[1†], Min-Keun Kim[2], Heng Bo Jiang[3], In-Woong Um[4*] and Yu-Mi Kim[4]

1 Department of Oral and Maxillofacial Surgery, Graduate School of Clinical Dentistry, Korea University, Seoul, Korea

2 Department of Oral and Maxillofacial Surgery, College of Dentistry, Gangneung-Wonju National University, Gangneung, Republic of Korea

3 Stomatological Materials Laboratory, School of Stomatology, Shandong First Medical University and Shandong Academy of Medical Science, Tai'an, China

4 R&D Institute, Korea Tooth Bank, Seoul, Republic of Korea

*Address all correspondence to: h-bmp@hanmail.net

† Both authors contributed equally.

References

[1] Muñoz MA, Garín-Correa C, González-Arriagada W, Quintela Davila X, Häberle P, Bedran-Russo A, et al. The adverse effects of radiotherapy on the structure of dental hard tissues and longevity of dental restoration. International Journal of Radiation Biology. 2020;96(7):910-8.

[2] Abou Neel EA, Aljabo A, Strange A, Ibrahim S, Coathup M, Young AM, et al. Demineralization-remineralization dynamics in teeth and bone. Int J Nanomedicine. 2016;11:4743-63.

[3] Pandya M, Diekwisch TGH. Enamel biomimetics-fiction or future of dentistry. Int J Oral Sci. 2019;11(1):8. Epub 2019/01/06.

[4] Margolis HC, Beniash E, Fowler CE. Role of Macromolecular Assembly of Enamel Matrix Proteins in Enamel Formation. Journal of Dental Research. 2006;85(9):775-93.

[5] Kumar GS. Orban's Oral Histology & Embryology2015. 458 p.

[6] Yahyazadehfar M, Bajaj D, Arola DD. Hidden contributions of the enamel rods on the fracture resistance of human teeth. Acta Biomater. 2013;9(1):4806-14. Epub 2012/10/02.

[7] Bechtle S, Habelitz S, Klocke A, Fett T, Schneider GA. The fracture behaviour of dental enamel. Biomaterials. 2010;31(2):375-84. Epub 2009/10/02.

[8] Deutsch D, Catalano-Sherman J, Dafni L, David S, Palmon A. Enamel matrix proteins and ameloblast biology. Connect Tissue Res. 1995;32(1-4):97-107. Epub 1995/01/01.

[9] Heritier M. Experimental induction of cementogenesis on the enamel of transplanted mouse tooth germs. Arch Oral Biol. 1982;27(2):87-97. Epub 1982/01/01.

[10] Brookes SJ, Robinson C, Kirkham J, Bonass WA. Biochemistry and molecular biology of amelogenin proteins of developing dental enamel. Arch Oral Biol. 1995;40(1):1-14. Epub 1995/01/01.

[11] Bansal AK, Shetty DC, Bindal R, Pathak A. Amelogenin: A novel protein with diverse applications in genetic and molecular profiling. J Oral Maxillofac Pathol. 2012;16(3):395-9. Epub 2012/12/19.

[12] Arola DD, Gao S, Zhang H, Masri R. The Tooth: Its Structure and Properties. Dent Clin North Am. 2017;61(4):651-68. Epub 2017/09/10.

[13] Elfallah HM, Bertassoni LE, Charadram N, Rathsam C, Swain MV. Effect of tooth bleaching agents on protein content and mechanical properties of dental enamel. Acta Biomater. 2015;20:120-8. Epub 2015/04/07.

[14] Yahyazadehfar M, Arola D. The role of organic proteins on the crack growth resistance of human enamel. Acta Biomater. 2015;19:33-45. Epub 2015/03/26.

[15] Zeichner-David M. Is there more to enamel matrix proteins than biomineralization? Matrix Biology. 2001;20(5):307-16.

[16] Wright JT, Li Y, Suggs C, Kuehl MA, Kulkarni AB, Gibson CW. The role of amelogenin during enamel-crystallite growth and organization in vivo. European journal of oral sciences. 2011;119 Suppl 1(Suppl 1):65-9.

[17] Deutsch D, Leiser Y, Shay B, Fermon E, Taylor A, Rosenfeld E, et al. The Human Tuftelin Gene and the

Expression of Tuftelin in Mineralizing and Nonmineralizing Tissues. Connective Tissue Research. 2002;43(2-3):425-34.

[18] Wang H, Tannukit S, Zhu D, Snead ML, Paine ML. Enamel Matrix Protein Interactions. Journal of Bone and Mineral Research. 2005;20(6):1032-40.

[19] Bosshardt DD. Biological mediators and periodontal regeneration: a review of enamel matrix proteins at the cellular and molecular levels. Journal of Clinical Periodontology. 2008;35(s8):87-105.

[20] Vallittu P. Non-Metallic Biomaterials for Tooth Repair and Replacement2013. 432 p.

[21] Sculean A, Windisch P, Döri F, Keglevich T, Molnár B, Gera I. Emdogain in regenerative periodontal therapy. A review of the literature. Fogorv Sz. 2007;100(5):220-32, 11-9.

[22] Gestrelius S, Lyngstadaas SP, Hammarström L. Emdogain – periodontal regeneration based on biomimicry. Clinical Oral Investigations. 2000;4(2):120-5.

[23] Esposito M, Grusovin MG, Papanikolaou N, Coulthard P, Worthington HV. Enamel matrix derivative (Emdogain®) for periodontal tissue regeneration in intrabony defects. Cochrane Database of Systematic Reviews. 2009(4).

[24] Nasr-Esfahani M, Fekri S. Alumina/TiO2/hydroxyapatite interface nanostructure composite filters as efficient photocatalysts for the purification of air. Reaction Kinetics, Mechanisms and Catalysis. 2012;107(1):89-103.

[25] Orsini G, Ruggeri Jr A, Mazzoni A, Nato F, Manzoli L, Putignano A, et al. A review of the nature, role, and function of dentin non-collagenous proteins. Part 1: proteoglycans and glycoproteins. Endodontic Topics. 2009;21(1):1-18.

[26] Linde A. Dentin matrix proteins: Composition and possible functions in calcification. The Anatomical Record. 1989;224(2):154-66.

[27] Le BQ, Nurcombe V, Cool SM, van Blitterswijk CA, de Boer J, LaPointe VLS. The Components of Bone and What They Can Teach Us about Regeneration. Materials (Basel). 2017;11(1):14.

[28] Orsini G, Ruggeri A, Jr., Mazzoni A, Papa V, Piccirilli M, Falconi M, et al. Immunohistochemical identification of type I and type III collagen and chondroitin sulphate in human pre-dentine: a correlative FEI-SEM/TEM study. Int Endod J. 2007;40(9):669-78.

[29] Bertassoni LE, Stankoska K, Swain MV. Insights into the structure and composition of the peritubular dentin organic matrix and the lamina limitans. Micron. 2012;43(2):229-36.

[30] Bertassoni LE, Orgel JP, Antipova O, Swain MV. The dentin organic matrix - limitations of restorative dentistry hidden on the nanometer scale. Acta Biomater. 2012;8(7):2419-33. Epub 2012/03/15.

[31] Breschi L, Maravic T, Cunha SR, Comba A, Cadenaro M, Tjäderhane L, et al. Dentin bonding systems: From dentin collagen structure to bond preservation and clinical applications. Dental Materials. 2018;34(1):78-96.

[32] Ravindran S, George A. Dentin Matrix Proteins in Bone Tissue Engineering. Adv Exp Med Biol. 2015;881:129-42.

[33] Butler WT. Dentin matrix proteins. Eur J Oral Sci. 1998;1:204-10.

[34] Delany AM, Amling M, Priemel M, Howe C, Baron R, Canalis E. Osteopenia

and decreased bone formation in osteonectin-deficient mice. J Clin Invest. 2000;105(7):915-23.

[35] Fisher LW, Fedarko NS. Six genes expressed in bones and teeth encode the current members of the SIBLING family of proteins. Connect Tissue Res. 2003;1:33-40.

[36] Ritchie H. The functional significance of dentin sialoprotein-phosphophoryn and dentin sialoprotein. International Journal of Oral Science. 2018;10(4):31.

[37] Duncan HF, Kobayashi Y, Shimizu E. Growth Factors and Cell Homing in Dental Tissue Regeneration. Curr Oral Health Rep. 2018;5(4):276-85. Epub 2019/02/02.

[38] Goustin AS, Leof EB, Shipley GD, Moses HL. Growth factors and cancer. Cancer Res. 1986;46(3):1015-29. Epub 1986/03/01.

[39] Chmilewsky F, Jeanneau C, Dejou J, About I. Sources of dentin-pulp regeneration signals and their modulation by the local microenvironment. J Endod. 2014;40(4 Suppl):S19-25. Epub 2014/04/05.

[40] Kim SG, Malek M, Sigurdsson A, Lin LM, Kahler B. Regenerative endodontics: a comprehensive review. Int Endod J. 2018;51(12):1367-88. Epub 2018/05/20.

[41] Kim SG, Zhou J, Solomon C, Zheng Y, Suzuki T, Chen M, et al. Effects of growth factors on dental stem/progenitor cells. Dent Clin North Am. 2012;56(3):563-75. Epub 2012/07/28.

[42] Mazzoni A, Breschi L, Carrilho M, Nascimento FD, Orsini G, Ruggeri Jr A, et al. A review of the nature, role, and function of dentin non-collagenous proteins. Part II: enzymes, serum proteins, and growth factors. Endodontic Topics. 2009;21(1):19-40.

[43] Mitsiadis TA, Rahiotis C. Parallels between tooth development and repair: conserved molecular mechanisms following carious and dental injury. J Dent Res. 2004;83(12):896-902.

[44] Magloire H, Romeas A, Melin M, Couble ML, Bleicher F, Farges JC. Molecular Regulation of Odontoblast Activity under Dentin Injury. Advances in Dental Research. 2001;15(1):46-50.

[45] Roberts-Clark DJ, Smith AJ. Angiogenic growth factors in human dentine matrix. Archives of Oral Biology. 2000;45(11):1013-6.

[46] Mohan S, Baylink DJ. Bone growth factors. Clin Orthop Relat Res. 1991(263):30-48. Epub 1991/02/01.

[47] Baylink DJ, Finkelman RD, Mohan S. Growth factors to stimulate bone formation. Journal of Bone and Mineral Research. 1993;8(S2):S565-S72.

[48] Shim KS. Pubertal growth and epiphyseal fusion. Ann Pediatr Endocrinol Metab. 2015;20(1):8-12. Epub 2015/04/18.

[49] Gual-Vaqués P, Polis-Yanes C, Estrugo-Devesa A, Ayuso-Montero R, Mari-Roig A, López-López J. Autogenous teeth used for bone grafting: A systematic review. Med Oral Patol Oral Cir Bucal. 2018;23(1):e112-e9. Epub 2017/12/24.

[50] Um I-W, Ku J-K, Kim Y-M, Yun P-Y, Chang N-H, Kim Y-K, et al. Allogeneic Demineralized Dentin Matrix Graft for Guided Bone Regeneration in Dental Implants. Applied Sciences. 2020;10(13):4661.

[51] Hwan Jung M, Hun Lee J, Wadhwa P, Bo Jiang H, Jang HS, Seok Lee E. Bone Regeneration in Peri-Implant Defect Using Autogenous Tooth Biomaterial

Enriched with Platelet-Rich Fibrin in Animal Model. Applied Sciences. 2020;10(6):1939.

[52] Lee Y-K, Wadhwa P, Cai H, Jung S-U, Zhao BC, Rim J-S, et al. Micro-CT and Histomorphometric Study of Bone Regeneration Effect with Autogenous Tooth Biomaterial Enriched with Platelet-Rich Fibrin in an Animal Model. Scanning. 2021;2021:6656791.

[53] Kim J-H, Wadhwa P, Cai H, Kim D-H, Zhao BC, Lim H-K, et al. Histomorphometric Evaluation of Socket Preservation Using Autogenous Tooth Biomaterial and BM-MSC in Dogs. Scanning. 2021;2021:6676149.

[54] Wadhwa P, Lee JH, Zhao BC, Cai H, Rim J-S, Jang H-S, et al. Microcomputed Tomography and Histological Study of Bone Regeneration Using Tooth Biomaterial with BMP-2 in Rabbit Calvarial Defects. Scanning. 2021;2021:6690221.

[55] Ku J-K, Um I-W, Jun M-K, Kim I-h. Dentin-Derived-Barrier Membrane in Guided Bone Regeneration: A Case Report. Materials. 2021;14(9):2166.

[56] Bartlett JD. Dental enamel development: proteinases and their enamel matrix substrates. ISRN Dent. 2013;16(684607):684607.

[57] Gil-Bona A, Bidlack FB. Tooth Enamel and its Dynamic Protein Matrix. Int J Mol Sci. 2020;21(12).

[58] Gadhia K, McDonald S, Arkutu N, Malik K. Amelogenesis imperfecta: an introduction. British Dental Journal. 2012;212(8):377-9.

[59] Wright JT, Hart TC, Hart PS, Simmons D, Suggs C, Daley B, et al. Human and Mouse Enamel Phenotypes Resulting from Mutation or Altered Expression of AMEL, ENAM, MMP20 and KLK4. Cells Tissues Organs. 2009;189(1-4):224-9.

[60] Simmer JP, Hu Y, Lertlam R, Yamakoshi Y, Hu JC. Hypomaturation enamel defects in Klk4 knockout/LacZ knockin mice. J Biol Chem. 2009;284(28):19110-21.

[61] Wright JT, Frazier-Bowers S, Simmons D, Alexander K, Crawford P, Han ST, et al. Phenotypic variation in FAM83H-associated amelogenesis imperfecta. J Dent Res. 2009;88(4):356-60.

[62] Carlson B. Human Embryology and Developmental Biology. 5th ed2013. 520 p.

[63] Kwon Hyuk-Jae Edward JR. Development of Teeth. : Elsevier; 2018 7-Feb-18.

[64] Chi BNDDDCAA. Color Atlas of Oral and Maxillofacial Diseases. 1 ed: Elsevier; 2018. 544 p.

[65] Williams R, Perez VA, Mangum JE, Hubbard MJ. Pathogenesis of Molar Hypomineralisation: Hypomineralised 6-Year Molars Contain Traces of Fetal Serum Albumin. Front Physiol. 2020;11(619).

[66] Perez VA, Mangum JE, Hubbard MJ. Pathogenesis of Molar Hypomineralisation: Aged Albumin Demarcates Chalky Regions of Hypomineralised Enamel. Frontiers in Physiology. 2020;11(1232).

[67] Babajko S, Jedeon K, Houari S, Loiodice S, Berdal A. Disruption of Steroid Axis, a New Paradigm for Molar Incisor Hypomineralization (MIH). Front Physiol. 2017;8(343).

[68] Williams R, Perez VA, Mangum JE, Hubbard MJ. Pathogenesis of Molar Hypomineralisation: Hypomineralised 6-Year Molars Contain Traces of Fetal Serum Albumin. Frontiers in Physiology. 2020;11(619).

[69] Almuallem Z, Busuttil-Naudi A. Molar incisor hypomineralisation

(MIH) – an overview. British Dental Journal. 2018;225(7):601-9.

[70] Wong MCM, Glenny AM, Tsang BWK, Lo ECM, Worthington HV, Marinho VCC. Topical fluoride as a cause of dental fluorosis in children. Cochrane Database of Systematic Reviews. 2010(1).

[71] Linda McManus RM. Pathobiology of Human Disease. 1 ed: Academic Press; 2014. 5000 p.

[72] DenBesten P, Li W. Chronic fluoride toxicity: dental fluorosis. Monogr Oral Sci. 2011;22:81-96.

[73] Sapir S, Shapira J. Dentinogenesis imperfecta: an early treatment strategy. Pediatr Dent. 2001;23(3):232-7.

Chapter 2

Fluoride and Other Trace Elements in Dental Hard Tissue

Y.B. Aswini, Vikrant Mohanty and Kavita Rijhwani

Abstract

Fluorides and other trace elements are a part of various biological and chemical responses in the human body. They collaboratively work with all proteins, enzymes, and co-enzymes to carry out the different functions and in redox reactions. The dietary substances may not have an adequate amount of these essential trace elements, resulting in the development of dental soft and hard tissue disorders associated with their deficiencies. To tackle this, dietary supplements will be needed. So, the current chapter has thoroughly addressed the importance of trace elements in dental hard tissues. This has also discussed the effect of fluoride and other trace elements on dental hard tissues, as there is limited literature available in this area. This will provide an overall understanding of how trace elements are an essential part and their importance in oral diseases control and prevention.

Keywords: trace elements, fluoride, dental structure, mechanism of action, distribution

1. Introduction

Carbon, hydrogen, and nitrogen elements make up about 96 percent of all living things. In the living system, nearly half of all recognized elements are present in detectable concentrations. The physiological activities of 23 elements are identified in humans and other mammals, 11 of which are categorized as trace elements (TEs) [1]. Vanadium, chromium, manganese (Mn), iron (Fe), cobalt, copper (Cu), zinc (Zn), and molybdenum are transition elements, while selenium (Se), fluorine, and iodine are non-metal elements [1, 2]. TEs, unlike sodium, calcium, magnesium, potassium, and chlorine, which are macronutrients that must be consumed in large quantities, are micronutrients that must be consumed in small amounts. (usually lower than 100 mg/day). Major and Minor TEs are both essential for human health. Due to natural or man-made causes, a lack or excess of these elements may have serious clinical implications [2].

A tooth's structure includes hard tissue (enamel, dentine, and cement) as well as soft tissue (pulp and periodontal ligaments). A tooth has a multicellular structure that can collaborate with the maxillofacial region functionally [2, 3].

Trace elements (TEs) are essential for human health. Toxic effects are caused by a lack of or an overabundance of TEs. TEs have a huge impact on both human and dental health. It is involved in the functions of essential biological polyphosphate compounds such as ATP, DNA, and RNA. In the tooth structure, TEs are found in various concentrations. Teeth are affected by changes in the density of certain TEs. Caries susceptibility is increased when the density of certain TEs is altered. Others function as a barrier to the development of caries. Zinc (Zn), phosphorus (P), and magnesium (Mg) are common TEs that have a significant impact on dental health. The use of tissue samplings such as blood, semen, teeth, nails, and hair to measure TE values in order to define and correct these effects has a significant impact. Teeth are widely regarded as a reliable indicator of TEs. As a result, TEs have a big impact on the development of healthy teeth [4].

2. Trace elements in dental hard tissues

The hard tissue that protects the tooth's surface is known as enamel. This layer's job is to protect the dentine-pulp complex. Enamel is the body's toughest and most resistant tissue. It's made up of 95–97% inorganic material (calcium hydroxyapatite crystals) and 1–2% organic material (proteins like amylogenic, enameline, ameloblastin, and tuftelin, to name a few), and 2–4% water [5]. TEs make up a small percentage of the 97 percent inorganic content and consists of Phosphorus (P-17%), calcium (Ca-36.5%), fluoride (F-0.016%), 3.0% carbon dioxide, 0.2% Na, 0.3% potassium (K), 0.016% Fluoride, 0.1% sulfur (S), 0.01% copper (Cu), 0.016% Zn, 0.003% silicon (Si); and low amounts of silver (Ag), strontium (Sr), barium (Ba), chromium (Cr), manganese (Mn), Vanadium (V). TE is deposited in human tooth enamel by the environment before and after the tooth's mineralization and maturation [6].

After Enamel, the next layer to the tooth is Dentin consists of an inorganic matrix 70% in weight (40–45% in volume) Organic matrix 20% by weight (30% in volume), and water 10% by weight (20–25% in volume). The organic portion consists of proteins like osteonectin, osteopontin, osteoclastin-like dentin Gla protein, dentin phosphorene, dentin matrix protein, and dentin sialoprotein and type I collagen fiber [6, 7]. The inorganic material consists of hydroxyapatite crystals and TEs (40 in number) which include Zn, Sr., Fe, Al, B, Ba, Pb having up to 1000 ppm concentration and Ni, Li, Ag, As, Se, Nb, Hg having 100 ppb concentration. An analysis of the relation with age of 10 trace elements in dentine found that boron (B), manganese (Mn), cobalt (Co), copper (Cu), zinc (Zn), rubidium (Rb), strontium (Sr), molybdenum (Mo), cadmium (Cd), and lead (Pb) and suggested that human dentine is an appropriate substance for relating sex and age [8].

3. Cementum

Cementum is a type of connective tissue that connects the periodontal ligament to the root surface and covers the root surface's outermost layer of calcite matrix [9]. Cement is a vascularized, mineralized tissue and has higher regeneration potential. It connects the dentin to the periodontal ligament and aids in the repair and regeneration of periodontal tissue after injury [10]. Cement's inorganic portion is identical to that of bone, dentin, and enamel.

The essential mineral part of cementum consists of calcium hydroxyapatite with amorphous calcium phosphate ($Ca10\ (PO4)\ 6\ (OH)\ 2$) and has a lower crystallinity than other calcifying tissues [11]. This lower crystallinity causes the cementum, to be easily decalcified and increases the tendency to absorb nearby ions like fluoride. That's why a higher concentration of fluoride is found in cementum ad compared to other parts of the tooth. In comparison to other calcifying tissues, the cement of adult mature teeth has higher fluoride content. The amount of magnesium in the cement is about half that of the dentin. In the deep layers of the cement, Mg levels gradually rise [9, 10].

4. Dental pulp

Dental pulp consists of Odontoblastfibroblast (collagen and elastic fibers forming cells), blood vessels, nerves, and lymphatic vessels that make up the tooth pulp that develops from the dental papilla [11]. The cells which are responsible for the formation of pre-dentin, dentin, and reparative dentin are Odontoblast [11]. When the pulp's health is threatened the pulp cells especially fibroblasts produce inflammatory mediators such as IL-8, IL-6, and vascular endothelial growth factors that are responsible for producing symptoms of pulp infection. The tooth pulp is responsible for a variety of biological functions, including nutrition, sensitivity, building, and defense. The health of the pulp is largely influenced by changes in blood pressure and arterial flow in the apical area. When tooth pulp is affected by stimulus or irritants like mechanical, chemical, thermal, or microbial agents causing vascular inflammatory responses like local tissue reactions and lymphatasis(affecting lymphatic drainage of pulp area) [12–14].

Dental caries is a microbiological infectious disease that causes the degradation of calcified tissues and the destruction of the organic part of the tooth leads to cavitation. The bacteria (from mutans Streptococci and Lactobacillus species), a susceptible tooth surface (host), and a nutrient (diet) to provide bacterial growth are all needed for the formation of dental caries. From enamel, caries progress to dentin and causes inflammation of the pulp [15, 16].

In a systematic review analysis of various studies assessing the role of trace elements in oral health, it was found that there are some trace elements that cause dental caries progression whereas certain trace elements may decrease the risk of developing dental caries [4].

The effects of fluoride and various trace elements on dental hard tissues are as follows:

1. **Fluoride as trace element**

Of the existing anticaries agents, fluoride is the most powerful and well-tested. Understanding the mechanism of fluoride's action in the prevention of dental caries is critical for developing the best fluoride delivery systems for optimal caries reduction. Although the exact and full mechanism of action of fluoride cannot be determined at this time, there is enough evidence to suggest that fluoride has a number of subtle effects on the calcium-phosphate system as well as the dental plaque metabolism. Fluorides can affect calcium-phosphate interactions in tooth enamel during the mineralization stage (before the tooth emerges) and, also, post eruptively by surface interactions with enamel, as well as during a carious attack [17, 18].

- **Mineral phase of enamel - a review**

Ca2+, PO43-, OH-, and carbonate are the key chemical components of tooth enamel ($CO3^{2-}$). These components are found in the form of microcrystals in enamel and dentin, and their spatial structure resembles that of the pure ternary mineral hydroxyapatite, Ca10(PO4)6(OH)2. Carbonate is a component of enamel's relatively large apatite crystals. Furthermore, teeth's mineral phase contains a variety of trace elements, the most significant of which is fluoride. Some of the elements are adsorbed on the surface of hydroxyapatite crystals, while others with the right size and charge will fill voids or replace calcium or phosphate in the crystal interior. As a result, it's obvious that enamel bioapatite is not pure apatite, but rather includes CO32-, Na+, Mg2+, F-, Sr2+, CI-, and other ions. Enamel apatite deviates from the stoichiometry of pure apatite in terms of Ca/P ratios due to a large number of substitutions in the crystal lattice. Enamel crystals also have a lot of flaws and are low in calcium and hydroxyl ions. The solubility of enamel tends to increase as voids and deviations from stoichiometry increase [19].

Fluoride incorporation within the apatite lattice has significant consequences. The formation of fluorapatite is caused by the replacement of hydroxyl groups by smaller fluoride ions, which causes a decrease in the dimension of the unit cell and has many effects on the physical and chemical properties of the crystals. Surface enamel (first 10 um) obtained from people living in fluoridated areas may contain 3000–4000 ppm of fluoride, whereas pure fluorapatite has a fluoride concentration of 38,000 ppm. It is clear that drinking fluoridated water causes just a small amount of fluoride ions to be substituted for hydroxyl ions, around 10%. Even this minor substitution appears to play a role in the strong cariostatic impact. The acquisition of fluoride by enamel is considered before exploring the mechanisms of fluoride action [19–22].

- **Acquisition of fluoride in enamel**

Fluoride enters dental enamel by two mechanisms: (1) systemically, through absorption of fluorides in water, drinks, foods, or fluoride supplements, and (2) topically, through oral fluids such as saliva, urine, plaque fluid, and topical fluoride solutions bathing enamel. Topical fluoride acquisition is limited to the enamel surface, mostly the first 10- to 30-pm layer, and is often limited to etched surfaces and incipient lesions.

- **Systemic acquisition of fluoride**

During the mineralization process, fluorides are introduced pre-eruptively into enamel from tissue fluid. The fluoride level acquired is determined by the fluoride concentration in the plasma, which is a feature of the fluoride consumed in water, food, or supplements. The fluoride concentration is relatively high during the early stages of enamel development, but it gradually decreases as the tooth matures and acquires more minerals [23].

During the pre-eruptively maturation period, when enamel undergoes rapid and more full mineralization, the majority of fluoride is incorporated into the sound surface of the enamel.

Since primary teeth have a shorter time of enamel maturation than permanent teeth, they absorb less fluoride. The slight variations in fluoride concentration between permanent teeth can also be explained by differences in tooth maturation time. In both fluoride and non-fluoride regions, a gradient concentration occurs with a declining concentration towards the dento-enamel junction in unerupted and erupted teeth [23].

While the majority of fluoride is acquired during the pre-eruptive growth of teeth, it is important to note that a large portion of the mineral component of enamel (about 10% in bovine enamel) is acquired during post-eruptive maturation [24].

Furthermore, the optimum value for enamel crystallinity is reached several years after the eruption. A significant amount of fluoride is introduced into surface enamel during this process of mineral deposition. Fluoride is less likely to disperse as teeth age and become more mineralized, so deposition is more limited to the surface. This causes a more pronounced fluoride concentration gradient, with lower concentrations towards the interior of enamel, though this is later decreased by abrasion on exposed areas of the tooth. The concentration of fluoride in populations that consumed water that was optimally fluoridated (1 ppm) during the development of the dentition is higher, Fluoride concentrations in total enamel of permanent teeth range from 200 to 300 ppm, with levels as high as 3000 ppm in the first 10 micrometer. The comparable fluoride concentration in non-fluoridated areas is about 150 ppm in whole enamel and under 2000 ppm in surface enamel. In the outer few micrometers of enamel, the gradient is very steep. These levels are lower in primary teeth, with fluoridated and non-fluoridated communities having 900 and 650 ppm in surface enamel, respectively [17, 25]. Fluoride concentration is the highest in surface enamel and decreases towards the inner parts. Fluoride concentrations in enamel vary from one surface to another on the same tooth. Fluoride concentrations in newly erupted tooth surface enamel are higher near the incisal edge than near the cervical margin [26]. However, after the eruption, subsequent wear and attrition of the enamel destroy the fluoride-rich outer enamel of the incisal edge at a faster rate than it is obtained, allowing it to fall below the cervical enamel.

Topical obtainment of fluoride is often acquired post-eruptively from the oral atmosphere in the enamel surface, but the accumulation is mostly limited to the surface. Foods, water, fluoride-containing beverages, toothpastes, mouth rinses, prophylactic pastes, topical solutions, and gels are all sources of fluoride.

- **Mechanisms of Cariostatic Action**

a. **Fluoride's Effect on Enamel Solubility**- It is widely accepted that caries are caused by bacterial acids demineralizing the mineral phase of the tooth. As a result, the solubility of tooth minerals may have an impact on the caries process. A potential mechanism by which fluoride decreases caries is by influencing the solubility of dental enamel, according to these claims. It is relatively easy to show that trace amounts of fluoride (−1 ppm) in an acid buffer solution significantly reduce enamel solubility, and that enamel readily acquires reduced solubility properties when exposed to a fluoride solution.

At pH 4.5, Ten Cate and Duijsters [27] found that 2 ppm F in a solution containing 2.2 mM Ca and P effectively prevented enamel demineralization. Proof that the slight rise of fluoride in enamel caused by drinking fluoridated water causes significant solubility differences is less conclusive.

Isaac et al. and Jenkins [28, 29] Solubility tests of intact enamel obtained from teeth of individuals living in fluoridated and non-fluoridated areas show a trend towards less solubility in the fluoridated classes. Moreno et al. [30] used apatites with well-defined levels of fluoride ranging from 0 to 3.4 percent to come to the conclusion that fluoride concentrations of 4000–8000 ppm were required to produce a significant decrease in enamel solubility. Fluoride concentrations in the molecular layers of surface enamel in fluoridated zones can be higher than those detected by the normal imprecise methods of collecting outer enamel. Explaining how a restricted substitution of fluoride ions for hydroxyl ions in enamel apatite can affect enamel solubility requires another consideration. Low levels of fluoride in the solution can react with the outer surfaces of dissolving hydroxyapatite crystals, forming a shell with fluorapatite solubility properties, according to Brown et al. [22].

The presence of small amounts of fluoride during a carious attack may therefore have a major impact on the properties of enamel crystals. This may explain why fluoride-containing products (dentifrices and mouth-rinses) are highly effective cariostatic agents when used on a regular or weekly basis for long periods of time. As previously stated, substitutions and defects cause enamel apatite to deviate from the stoichiometry of pure hydroxyapatite. Fluoride stabilizes the crystal structure of enamel, while carbonate and sodium increase its solubility and reactivity. Also, Nikiforuk et al. [31] found some evidence that the presence of fluoride during enamel production results in lower carbonate content. The dissolved enamel crystals preferentially lose carbonate during an incipient carious assault. Crystals containing less carbonate are thought to have lower reactivity and solubility, making them more resistant to caries. Fortunately, as the plaque's pH rises, recrystallization occurs, resulting in the formation of larger, more resistant crystals. The sum of these results is that fluoride has a slight but important effect on enamel solubility, even at the relatively low concentrations found in enamel.

a. **Effect of fluoride on mineral phase crystal structure** -As calcium phosphate precipitates from a saturated solution in the physiological pH range, the initial phase stoichiometry is typically less than the calcium/phosphate molar ratio (1.67) found in pure hydroxy-apatite. Brown et al. [22] found evidence that the initially formed solid phase is octacalcium phosphate, tricalcium phosphate, dicalcium phosphate, or a combination. The initial precipitate may also be an amorphous solid with no set calcium/phosphate ratio, according to some theories. Whatever the initial phase was like, it was transformed into hydroxyapatite and possibly some fluorapatite, the thermodynamically more stable phases under physiological conditions. Amjad and Nancollas [19] verified earlier work that fluoride at concentrations of 1–5 ppm enhanced the precipitation of the less soluble phase of calcium phosphate in very careful kinetic studies of calcium phosphate precipitation in the presence of fluoride ions. In the absence of fluoride, the phase that evolved first had the same stoichiometry as octacalcium phosphate. The Ca/P ratio of the solid phase increased in the presence of fluoride and matched that of fluorapatite. Evidence suggests that fluoride acts as a catalyst during mineralization, causing the more soluble precursor phases to transform into the thermodynamically more stable apatite. This in vitro process is active during tooth mineralization, as shown by the lower carbonate levels in enamel from fluoridated areas. Fluoride also favors the creation of more acid-resistant crystals during the demineralization-remineralization episodes that characterize carious attacks. Fluoride can be believed to stabilize the crystal structure of enamel apatite because of its ability to form a more stable apatite phase. It should be remembered that the lattice comprises columns of hydroxyl ions that are electrostatically bound to calcium ions. Some of the hydroxyl ions are still absent, and these vacancies reduce the crystal's stability. Fluorides may fill these voids or act as a hydroxyl group replacement, forming a stronger bond to the lattice site than hydroxyl ions. The negatively charged fluoride forms a tight hydrogen bond with the oxygen atom of the adjacent hydroxyl groups. Additionally, the better match of fluoride ions between calcium ions increases the electrostatic attraction between fluorides and calcium, further stabilizing the structure. While this argument has not been corroborated, the fluoride ions' strategic location may also prevent diffusion along the linear chain. Although this assertion has not been corroborated in synthetic hydroxyapatite with hydroxyl deficiencies similar to those found in enamel [Verbeeck et al.] [32], the strategic location of the fluoride ions can also obstruct diffusion along the linear chain. As a consequence of a small fluoride substitution in the lattice structure, the crystallinity and stability of the crystal are increased.

b. **Effect of fluoride on enamel remineralization**- Clinical remineralization and reversal of early carious lesions have been demonstrated experimentally in vivo [von der Fehr et al., 1970] and clinically observed [33]. Several researchers have recorded that fluorides improve this natural process in vitro [34, 35]. Salivary components and fluoride are now recognized as effective natural protection mechanism that allows enamel to respond to cariogenic challenges. In vitro, adding 0.05 mM fluoride to calcium phosphate solutions used to remineralize partially demineralized enamel increases the rate of remineralization by 4- to 8-fold [36]. In comparison to natural plaque, which has high fluoride levels, etched enamel remineralization results in higher fluoride levels in the enamel. This is referred to as enamel's adaptative response to the acidic environment in a specific area [37]. The minerals that form during remineralization are less soluble than those that form in the same solution but do not contain fluorides.

An important reservoir of fluoride is surface enamel from which fluoride is released during the demineralization phase of a carious attack. Fluoride ions are also released from plaque when the pH falls which may contribute to remineralization. The process of remineralization can function at the earliest stage of caries formation, i.e. when the first acid attack occurs.

As the pH starts to grow after the acid attack, fluoride in the microenvironment will trigger enamel dissolution to stop sooner. If the pH increases, fresh, bigger, less soluble crystals form, containing more fluoride, such as fluoridated hydroxyapatite, and less carbonate like fluoridated hydroxyapatite. The enamel is partially remineralized as a result of the procedure. Following exposure to fluoride, saliva, or plaque fluid, the amount of new minerals at the site may increase even more. When fluoride is applied at a later stage of caries growth, such as when a white spot is apparent, fluoride penetrates the surface layer and is absorbed preferentially by the porous sponge like the body of the lesion. This also decreases the solubility of the lesion, making it more vulnerable to acid attacks in the future. On radiographs prepared from thin parts taken through the lesion, successive fluoride exposures and caries attacks often result in a laminated appearance [38]. According to in vitro remineralization tests, the entire body of the white spot lesion does not need to be remineralized to become covered. If only the surface zone of a lesion is remineralized, the lesion can be stopped. When lesions are subjected to re-mineralizing solutions containing relatively high amounts of fluoride or calcium, this is easily accomplished [34]. As a result, the appearance of natural caries white spots in the mouth does not always imply that the region is actually under attack by caries. It may actually signify a region that has been attacked but is now partly remineralized and arrested as a result. Because of the absorption of organic stains, long-standing arrested lesions often appear as brown spots [35].

Because of the buffering effect of saliva and plaque, as well as the high concentrations of calcium and phosphate present, the caries process is complex, with periods of demineralization when plaque pH are minimal, alternating with periods of remineralization as pH rises. If the process is to be pushed in the direction of remineralization, the presence of trace amounts of fluorides released from enamel or normally present in plaque fluid is important [39]. This is a key mechanism by which fluoride decreases the incidence of caries.

c. **Effect of fluoride and tooth morphology** - Fluoride intake can affect the size and morphology of teeth in humans and laboratory animals. Most studies show that if fluoride is present during tooth development, diameters and cusp depths are smaller [40]. Such morphological modifications would help to reduce caries vulnerability by making teeth more self-cleaning, but it's unclear if the effects of optimal fluoride intake are substantial enough to be clinically significant.

Other trace elements (strontium and molybdenum) have similar effects in rats, raising questions about the fluoride effect's specificity. According to Aasenden and Peebles [18], molars. Molars in subjects who consumed fluoridated water or nutrients had shallower fissures and less carious lesions than molars in a non-fluoride control sample, according to Aasenden and Peebles [18], corroborating other clinical impressions. Deep fissures collect more plaque and are more difficult to clean than shallow fissures. The improved morphology of the occlusal surface may be partly to blame for the lower level of occlusal caries observed in fluoridated areas, despite the fact that it is the least affected.

5. Distribution of trace elements other than fluoride in dental hard tissue and its mechanism of action

As per the various literature, it has been found that various trace elements have different roles in causing and preventing dental caries like Selenium, Cadmium, Magnesium, Platinum, Lead and Silicon are caries promoting elements whereas other than Fluoride, Phosphorus, Molybdenum Vanadium, Strontium and Lithium are cariostatic elements.

The effects of trace elements on oral dental tissues are as follows-.

5.1 Vanadium (V)

The vanadium is found with industrial resources such as oil refineries and power plants. The majority of food compounds contain lesser concentrations whereas Seafood has a higher concentration of Vanadium and daily uptake from all source's ranges from 0.01–0.02 mg [41].

Various studies have been done to assess the role of Vanadium in the development of prevention of dental caries. It's found to be caries protective in animal studies and studies on rats but on the contrary studies on monkeys when they drank water with Vanadium content tend to have more carious lesions in their mouth. So exact role in the prevention and development of caries is still not clear [4].

5.2 Strontium (SR)

Strontium is universally present in the environment. Though it is non-essential but still present in all living beings. This element bears a resemblance to Calcium as it has a tendency to be taken by bones and skeleton. Depending upon the amount received, it can have beneficial and harmful effects on humans [42].

Strontium is considered to be caries protective as per the literature. The strontium makes the enamel more stable and stronger as compared to pure calcium content. It also found that remineralized process in enamel with strontium in solution easier and faster as compared to without strontium solution and because of this the tooth enamel stable and more resistant to caries and acid attack [43].

The epidemiological studies suggest that high strontium content is associated with decreased carious lesions or good enamel. The strontium content decrease with age and is found to be more young as compared to older people.

5.3 Lithium (Li)

Lithium has an inverse relation with the development of dental caries. Various studies reported with reduced incidence of caries in presence of lithium in humans [4]. Mostly the lithium exposure occurs with drinking water and if in excess can have an effect on different tissues or organs in animals like affects the thyroid function and also causes histopathological changes in salivary glands [44]. It has medicinal use in various psychiatric disorders like bipolar disorders [45].

5.4 Copper (Cu)

Copper is a component of a variety of metalloenzymes that act as oxidases to reduce molecular oxygen. Adult men and women should consume 900 g of fiber per day. Copper intake from food is approximately 1.0 to 1.6 mg/day for adult men and women in the United States. Adults have a Tolerable Upper Intake Level (UL) of 10,000 g/day (10 mg/day), a value based on protection from liver damage as the critical adverse effect. Greater amounts of copper are found in seafood, green leafy vegetables, animal products, pulses, and grains [46].

Oral Health and Diseases: What Role Does It Play- Hypochromic anemia, neutropenia, hypopigmentation of hair and skin, irregular bone structure with skeletal fragility and osteoporosis, joint pain, reduced immunity, vascular aberrations, and kinky hair are all signs of copper deficiency [47].

- If a person has copper deficiency for a long-time during stages of active growth it can cause anemia and abnormal keratinization of oral soft tissues. Reduced iron oxidation and decreased ferroxidase activity of ceruloplasmin are responsible for the anemic impact [48].

- Infections: Due to the accompanied neutropenia, lowered immunity can result in a variety of oral infections [49]. Granulocyte maturation disorder has been observed in the bone marrow, as well as vacuolation in neutrophils.

- Bone defects and pain due to abnormal functioning of ascorbate and lysyl oxidase leads to osteoporosis like changes in the body i.e. lack of trabecular pattern and cortex thinning.

- Oral lesions: according to several reports, the average serum copper levels were present in the Sera from patients with oral potentially malignant conditions like oral leukoplakia and oral submucous fibrosis, as well as malignant tumors like squamous cell carcinoma, and was substantially higher.

- The average copper intake in India is 2.1–3.9 mg/day, but it is more than 5 mg/day due to areca nut chewing. Copper released from areca nuts during chewing is thought to come into direct contact with the oral epithelium and be dissolved in saliva. Copper is said to be found in saliva for up to 30 minutes. The longer copper is present in saliva, the more likely it is to be absorbed by the oral epithelium [48]. Copper occurs in the blood after 15 minutes of ingestion of areca nut and its ingredients, according to some [50]. Cu serum levels steadily rise in patients with oral submucous fibrosis as the condition progresses clinically. However, the local impact of increased salivary copper levels may be more significant than the increased serum levels. Other schools of thought attributed a decrease in copper serum concentrations to copper's role in upregulating lysyl oxidase, which resulted in excessive collagen cross-linking [51].

- Cu is also thought to have a caries-promoting effect [52].

5.5 Selenium (Se)

Selenium salts are essential for a variety of cellular functions in the human body, but too much of them is toxic [53]. It is present in the liver, kidneys, seafood, poultry, grains, grain oils, milk, fruits, and vegetables, and a maximum intake of 70 micrograms is recommended [54]. It is required for the formation of anti-oxidants enzymes in the body.

Selenium is a non-metallic substance that occurs naturally and is absorbed by the body through food or inhalation. Intake of selenium was linked to an increase in dental caries. It has been stated that selenium settles in the enamel's micro-crystal structure at the start of decay, making it more susceptible to dissolution [54].

Furthermore, a reduction in selenium levels in the body has been linked to oxidative stress. According to a new study, patients who developed oral mucositis as a result of high-dose chemotherapy significantly shortened the duration and severity of the condition and also has cytoprotective impact and antiulcer activity on subsequent reinforcement [55].

5.6 Manganese (MN)

The amount of manganese in food varies greatly. Peanuts and grains have the highest concentrations, while milk products, meat, poultry, fish, and sea products have the lowest. Manganese can also be present in coffee and tea, which account for 10% of daily intake. On average, an adult's body contains 15 mg of manganese, which is often found in nucleic acid. The regular requirement is between 2 and 5 milligrams. Manganese is a component of metalloenzymes and acts as an enzyme activator. Manganese concentrations range from 0.3 to 2.9 ug manganese/g in all mammalian tissues. Tissues with a lot of mitochondria and pigments (like the retina and dark skin) have a lot of manganese concentrations in them.

Manganese is a TE that can be ingested by food, air, or water and incorporated into the enamel. Furthermore, Mn has the ability to change Ca′s position at HAP. Mn can be used in synthetic HAP without degrading the crystal area size, according to several studies [56].

Manganese concentrations are normally higher in bones, livers, pancreas, and kidneys than in other tissues. The bones are the most valuable manganese shop. Manganese is one of 49 elements found in enamel hydroxyapatite crystals, and it is normally present in very small amounts. Manganese concentrations in enamel range from 0.08 to 20 ppm, or 0.08–20 mg/kg, and in dentine from 0.6 to 1000 ppm. The concentration of Mn is higher in permanent dentition compared to primary dentition [57].

Manganese is being increasingly linked to the occurrence of tooth decay. According to one study, the incidence of dental caries in males increased in areas with higher manganese content. As a result, it is stressed that manganese promotes caries [4].

5.7 Zinc (ZN)

Zinc is found in the human body in amounts ranging from 2 to 4 grams. The prostate, eyeballs, brain, muscles, bones, kidney, and liver all store zinc. It is the only metal used in all enzyme groups and is the second most common transition metal in species after iron. The concentration of Zn in plasma (10%) remains constant even when intake is higher and in plasma 60% is tightly bound to albumin and the rest to transferrin (40%) [58, 59].

The RDA of Zinc is 15–20 mg. The pancreas and intestines excrete approximately 2–5 mg per day. Pregnancy, loss of liquid, oral contraceptive use, blood loss, and acute infection all having lower plasma zinc levels.

Zinc is needed for cell reproduction, differentiation, and metabolic functions. Zinc also aids normal development during pregnancy, infancy, and adolescence [60, 61]. Zinc is present primarily in animal products such as beef, milk, and fish. Phytonutrients are poor in zinc bio adjustment [58].

Oral Health and Diseases: What role does it play?

1. Zinc is present in the oral cavity i.e. in Enamel, Dentin, and Plaque (Naturally present). Oral health products containing zinc are used to regulate plaque, minimize odor, and delay the development of calculus. Following delivery from mouth rinses and toothpaste, zinc elevated concentrations in plaque and saliva can be retained for long periods of time. Despite the fact that low concentrations of zinc can both minimize enamel demineralization and alter remineralization, the anti-cariogenic efficacy is still debatable and contradicted by numerous studies [62].

2. Taste disorders: Zinc plays an important role in taste functions at different stages of organization, including taste buds, taste sense nerve transmission, and anatomical structures like the brain. Early researchers concluded that taste disruptions are caused by zinc deficiency due to some etiology, and therefore zinc depletion is still corrected for patients reporting taste imbalances [63].

3. A rodent study found that a zinc-deficient diet can cause parakeratosis of the normally ortho-keratinized oral mucosa. As a result, zinc deficiency can be a risk factor for periodontal and oral diseases and causes parakeratosis in soft oral mucosa like in cheeks, tongue, and food pipe [64].

4. Act as a cofactor for superoxide dismutase enzyme and zinc deficiency is a finding of patients with potentially premalignant lesions such as oral leukoplakia that could be due to more intake of zinc in reaction to higher copper found in arecanut and oxidants produced during tobacco usage [65, 66].

5. In contrast to common opinion, limited evidence indicates that zinc has a carcinogenic effect [67].

5.8 Cadmium (Cd)

Cadmium accumulates in the liver and bones as soon as it reaches the body and is released slowly (cadmium reference). It causes a major environmental issue as a result of being received by plants and entering the food chain, or as a result of being washed from the soil and hitting the water environment. Furthermore, chelating agents accelerate the downward carriage of cadmium from the soil, which can contribute to contamination of drinking and irrigation waters as it reaches underground water bodies [68, 69].

Exposure to cadmium has been linked to a number of health problems, including kidney failure and skeletal problems, and heart diseases [70]. It can be released from dentures and materials containing metal alloys in the mouth (rigidly bound with metallothioneins) and can accumulate in teeth and other oral tissues.

Cadmium has been linked to an increase in the occurrence of tooth decay. However, it is said that cadmium settlement in teeth after growth is ineffective in preventing caries. According to some animal studies, there is a clear connection between the formation of dental caries and cadmium intake during the dental growth period [4]. The power of increased exposure to and diffusion of this toxic material on the general and oral health of vulnerable populations such as children is fetching increasingly significant [4].

5.9 Lead (Pb)

Lead may be consumed by tainted food and beverages as a result of industrial activity [51]. Lead enters the food chain through vegetables grown in polluted soil, for example. Lead can be transferred from polluted soil to plants and grass, potentially resulting in toxic metal accumulation in vegetating ruminants, especially cattle. Lead accumulation causes toxic effects in animals, as well as toxic effects in people who drink toxic metal-contaminated meat and milk [71].

It is a radioactive metal that is harmful to the human body. At the HAP of teeth, lead has the potential to translocate with Ca + 2 and resulting in decreasing the size of hydroxyapatite crystals [72].

In the atmosphere or diet, lead is passed to body hard tissues such as teeth and might be having an effect on increasing dental caries. Furthermore, it has been discovered that lead promotes the development of enamel hypoplasia. As per the literature, it shows have a probable connection between increasing lead levels in saliva and the formation of dental caries in children with early tooth decay. As a result, lead is critical in the formation of new caries lesions [4, 72, 73].

5.10 Iron (Fe)

Iron (Fe) is abundant in nature and a biologically important part of all living organisms, unlike other TE. Regardless of geological abundance, when oxygen comes into contact with iron, it forms hardly soluble oxides. As a result, it is poorly absorbed by species [74].

Iron is found in liver, beef, poultry products, and fish, as well as cereals, green leafy vegetables, pulses, nuts, oilseeds, and dried fruits. Iron, as an important nutrient, is primarily absorbed by green vegetables. Enamel has been found to have low iron concentrations [75]. RDA ranges from 4 to 5 gm and is essential to maintain a healthy body.

6. Detection of trace elements and assessment of nutritional status

This was done as follows:

a. Despite the fact that different methods have been used to assess the existence of trace elements, due to their large distribution within living tissues and enzyme systems, it is a time-consuming and fruitless task. To determine the sum of trace elements, colorimetric and spectrographic methods are widely used. For solitary element analysis, spectroscopy and electrochemical methods are typically used, while for multiple-element analysis, neutron activation analysis and spectroscopic methods are typically used [76].

b. Iron deficiency can be easily diagnosed routinely by laboratory test like Complete blood count with having the high total iron-binding capability, a low serum iron level, and a low serum ferritin concentration. The erythrocyte zinc porphyrin assay, has recently been used in primary screening for determining iron status [77, 78].

c. The optimum copper-zinc plasma or serum ratio has been stated to be 0.70–1.00. As previously mentioned in the report, diagnosing zinc deficiency is a difficult task. The most popular indices for measuring zinc deficiency are plasma or serum zinc levels [79, 80].

d. Since tissue chromium stores do not appear to accurately represent blood chromium, serum chromium concentration is not an accurate measure of chromium status. The existence of an extreme chromium deficiency is thought to be indicated by serum chromium levels less than 0.14–0.15 ng/mL. A person's serum chromium level may be elevated as a result of excessive chromium exposure from work or an accident.

e. The nutritional status of selenium has been determined using various tissues such as blood, hair, and nails. In general, if dietary selenium consumption is consistent, these tissues may provide a reliable assessment of selenium status.

f. It is difficult to assess the status of other trace elements in typical individuals' tissue levels.

7. Sources of trace elements

The location of trace elements on dental hard tissue like enamel and dentin may differ and also within the structure. The Cu, Pb, Co, Al, I, Sr., Se, Ni, and Mn more on enamel whereas Fe and F more on dentin and cementum.

Also, within the enamel, the outer surface has more Iron, Lead, and Manganese than inside layers suggesting that mostly these come from the external environment and get deposited on tooth enamel after an eruption or during calcification.

Trace elements can reach the human body through a variety of routes, including food, water, and air. Dental materials and fluids (such as saliva, dental prosthesis, and dental porcelain) are discussed below as potential sources of trace elements in tooth enamel [81].

a. **Saliva** - Saliva is actively washing teeth. The structure of the enamel surface is considered to be affected by many trace elements present in saliva. It varies among the population and in a great amount the trace elements found in enamel and also found in saliva (Na, Mg, K, and Zn). The amount of trace elements in one's saliva varies from person to person. The most abundant trace elements in saliva are also the most abundant trace elements in tooth enamel (Na, Mg, K, and Zn and it suggests that saliva can have a profound effect on enamel demineralization and remineralization.

b. **Dental prostheses** - Partial dentures can be a source of trace elements discovered in teeth. Patients with partial dentures have higher levels of Cr, Co, Fe, and Ni in their saliva than patients without partial dentures. As a result, the accumulation of trace elements in tooth enamel can be affected by the presence of dentures in the mouth. The effect of trace elements presents in dental prostheses on tooth enamel will be confirmed in future studies.

c. **Dental porcelain** - This material consists of a glass matrix and a leucite crystallite phase. It contains minerals like Si (57–66%), B (15–25%), Al (7–15%), Na (7–12%), K (7–15%), and Li (0.5–3%). The concentrations of these elements in tooth enamel were found to be closely associated. This finding suggests that dental porcelain may be another potential source of these elements in tooth enamel but need to confirm with future studies.

8. Conclusion

Though trace elements are only needed in trace amounts, their optimal presence is critical for the body's normal physiological functioning and for upholding the body's biodynamics. Excess and deficiency both contribute to the onset, development, and promotion of different disease processes. As a result, having a thorough understanding of these trace elements is critical for disease prevention and optimum health.

Nutritional and clinical diagnosis of trace element defects is one of the most daunting activities. Deficient intake of an important trace element can cause significant biological functions within tissues to be harmed, and restoring physiological levels of that element can restore or prevent that function from being harmed. The amount of main trace metals circulating in the blood and deposited in cells is controlled and regulated by an intricate mechanism in the human body. When the body fails to function properly or there are inappropriate levels in dietary sources, excessive levels of these trace elements may develop. A diet rich in antioxidants and essential minerals is essential for a healthy mind and body, according to numerous lines of proof. In recent years, preventive medicine has gotten more coverage than anything else, as the adage goes, "prevention is better than cure." Oral and general health are inextricably linked, and the oral cavity can effectively reflect systemic health. Oral diseases such as oral leukoplakia, oral submucous fibrosis, oral cancer, and others have been treated with a mixture of micronutrients and trace elements because their combined effect is more effective than a single application. As a result, general and oral healthcare professionals must be familiar with the clinical aspects of trace elements.

Author details

Y.B. Aswini*, Vikrant Mohanty and Kavita Rijhwani
Department of Public Health Dentistry, Maulana Azad Institute of Dental Sciences, New Delhi

*Address all correspondence to: phdaswini@gmail.com

References

[1] Fraga CG. Relevance, essentiality and toxicity of trace elements in human health. Molecular Aspects of Medicine. 2005;**26**(4-5):235-244

[2] Brown CJ, Chenery SR, Smith B, Mason C, Tomkins A, Roberts GJ, et al. Environmental influences on the trace element content of teeth implications for disease and nutritional status. Archives of Oral Biology. 2004;**49**:705-717

[3] Dogan MS, Yavas MC, Yavuz Y, Erdogan S, Yener İ, Simsek İ, et al. Effect of electromagnetic fields and antioxidants on the trace element content of rat teeth. Drug Design, Development and Therapy. 2017;**11**:1393-1398

[4] Pathak MU, Shetty V, Kalra D. Trace elements and oral health: A systematic review. Journal of Advanced Oral Research. 2016;7(2):12-20

[5] Robinson C, Weatherell JA, Hallsworth AS. Variation in composition of dental enamel within thin ground tooth sections. Caries Research. 1971;**5**:44-57. DOI: 10.1159/000259731

[6] Goldberg M, Kulkarni AB, Young M, Boskey A. Dentin: Structure, composition and mineralization. Frontiers in Bioscience (Elite Edition). 2011;**1**(3):711-735

[7] Shashikiran ND, Subba Reddy VV, Hiremath MC. Estimation of trace elements in sound and carious enamel of primary and permanent teeth by atomic absorption spectrophotometry: An in vitro study. Indian Journal of Dental Research. 2007;**18**:157-162

[8] Fernández-Escudero AC, Legaz I, Prieto-Bonete G, et al. Aging and trace elements in human coronal tooth dentine. Scientific Reports. 2020;**10**: 9964. DOI: 10.1038/s41598-020-66472-1

[9] Tziafas D. Composition and structure of cementum: Strategies for bonding. In: Eliades G, Watts D, Eliades T, editors. Dental Hard Tissues and Bonding. Berlin/Heidelberg: Springer; 2005. pp. 177-193

[10] Papagerakis P, Mitsiadis T. Development and structure of teeth and periodontal tissues. In: Primer on the Metabolic Bone Diseases and Disorders of Mineral Metabolism. 8th ed. New York: John Wiley & Sons; 2013

[11] Ten Cate AR. Oral Histology. Development, Structure and Function. 5th ed. St. ed. Louis: Mosby; 1998

[12] Hsieh SC, Tsao JT, Lew WZ, Chan YH, Lee LW, Lin CT, et al. Static magnetic field attenuates lipopolysaccharide-induced inflammation in pulp cells by affecting cell membrane stability. Scientific World Journal. 2015:492683

[13] Han G, Hu M, Zhang Y, Jiang H. Pulp vitality and histologic changes in human dental pulp after the application of moderate and severe intrusive orthodontic forces. American Journal of Orthodontics and Dentofacial Orthopedics. 2013;**144**(4):518-522

[14] Doğan MS, Yavaş MC, Günay A, Yavuz İ, Deveci E, Akkuş Z, et al. The protective effect of melatonin and Ganoderma lucidum against the negative effects of extremely low frequency electric and magnetic fields on pulp structure in rat teeth. Biotechnology and Biotechnological Equipment. 2017;**31**(5):979-988

[15] Kutsch VK. Dental caries: An updated medical model of risk assessment. The Journal of Prosthetic Dentistry. 2014;**111**(4):280-285

[16] Fontana M, Young DA, Wolff MS. Evidence-based caries, risk assessment,

and treatment. Dental Clinics of North America. 2009;**53**(1):149-161

[17] Aasenden R, Moreno EC, Brudevold F. Fluoride levels in the surface of different types of human teeth. Archives of Oral Biology. 1973;**18**:1403

[18] Aasenden R, Peebles TC. Effects of fluoride supplementation from birth on human deciduous and permanent teeth. Archives of Oral Biology. 1974;**19**:321

[19] Amjad Z, Nancollas GH. Effect of fluoride on the growth of hydroxylapatite and human dental enamel. Caries Research. 1979;**13**:250

[20] Birkeland JM, Charlton G. Effect of pH on the fluoride ion activity of plaque. Caries Research. 1976;**10**:72

[21] Briner WW, Gray JA, Francis MD. Significance of enamel remineralization. Journal of Dental Research. 1974;**53**:239

[22] Brown WE, Gregory TM, Chow LC. Effects of fluoride on enamel solubility and cariostasis. Caries Research. 1977;**11**(suppl. 1):118

[23] Weatherell JA, Deutsch D, Robinson C, Hallsworth AS. Assimilation of fluoride by enamel throughout the life of the tooth. Caries Research. 1977;**11**(suppl. 1):85

[24] Sakae, T.: Hirai, G. Calcification and crystallization in bovine enamel. Journal of Dental Research. 1982;**61**:57

[25] Tinanoff N, Wei SHY, Parkins FM. Effect of a pumice prophylaxis on fluoride uptake in tooth enamel. Journal of the American Dental Association. 1974;**88**:384

[26] Weatherell JA, Deutsch D, Robinson C, Hallsworth AS. Assimilation of fluoride by enamel throughout the life of the tooth. Caries Research. 1977;**11**(suppl. 1):85

[27] Ten Cate JM, Duijsters IM. Influence of fluoride in solution on tooth demineralization. II. Microradiographic data. Caries Research. 1983;**17**:513

[28] Isaac S, Brudevold F, Smith FA, Gardner DE. Solubility rate and natural fluoride content of surface and subsurface enamel. Journal of Dental Research. 1958;**37**:254

[29] Jenkins GN. Theories on the mode of action of fluoride in reducing dental decay. Journal of Dental Research. 1963;**42**:445

[30] Moreno EC, Kresak M, Zahradnik RT. Physiochemical aspects of fluoride apatite systems relevant to the study of dental caries. Caries Research. 1977;**11**(suppl. 1):142

[31] Nikiforuk G, McLeod IM, Burgess RC, Grainger RM, Brown HK. Fluoride-carbonate relationships in dental enamel. Journal of Dental Research. 1962;**41**:1477

[32] Verbeeck RMH, Driessens FCM, Schaeken HG, Heijligers HJM. Diffusion inhibition as a mechanism for the caries-reducing effect of fluoride. Caries Research. 1980;**14**:311

[33] Grindahl H-G. Radiographic caries diagnosis. A study of caries progression and observer performance. Swedish Dental Journal. 1979;(suppl. 3)

[34] Silverstone LM, Wefel JS, Zimmerman BH, Clarkson BH, Featherstone MI. Remineralization of natural and artificial lesions in human dental enamel in vitro. Effect of calcium concentration of the calcifying fluid. Caries Research. 1981;**15**:138

[35] Featherstone JDB, Cutress TW, Rodgers BE, Dennison PJ. Remineralization of artificial caries-like lesions in vivo by a self-administered mouthrinse or paste. Caries Research. 1982;**16**:235

[36] Koulourides T, Ceuto H, Pigman W. Rehardening of softened enamel surfaces of human teeth by solutions of calcium phosphates. Nature (London). 1961;**189**:226

[37] Feagin FF, Patel PR, Koulourides T, Pigman W. Study of the effect of calcium, phos-phate, fluoride and hydrogen ion concentrations on the remineralization of partially demineralized human and bovine enamel surfaces. Archives of Oral Biology. 1971;**16**:535

[38] Weatherell JA, Robinson C, Hallsworth AS. Micro-analytical studies on single sections of enamel. In: Stack, Fearnhead, Tooth Enamel. Vol. 2. Bristol: Wright & Sons; 1971. p. 31

[39] Silverstone LM. Remineralization phenomena. Caries Research. 1977;**11**(suppl. 1):59

[40] Ten Cate JM, Buzalaf MAR. Fluoride mode of action: Once there was an observant dentist. Journal of Dental Research. 2019;**98**(7):725-730. DOI: 10.1177/0022034519831604

[41] US Department of Health and Human Services. Toxicological Profile for Vanadium. 2012

[42] Höllriegl V, München HZ. Strontium in the environment and possible human health effects. In: Nriagu JO, editor. Encyclopedia of Environmental Health. Burlington: Elsevier; 2011. pp. 268-275

[43] Prashanth L, Kattapagari KK, Chitturi RT, Baddam VRR, Prasad LK. A review on role of essential trace elements in health and disease. Journal Dr. NTR University of Health Sciences. 2015;**4**(2):75-78

[44] Özcan I. The histopathologic effects of lithium on rat salivary glands. ACTA Pharmaceutica Sciencia. 2000;**42**(4):107-111

[45] Usuda K, Kono K, Dote T, Watanabe M, Shimizu H, Tanimoto Y, et al. An overview of boron, lithium, and strontium in human health and profiles of these elements in urine of Japanese. Environmental Health and Preventive Medicine. 2007;**12**(6):231-237

[46] Institute of Medicine (US) Panel on Micronutrients. Dietary Reference Intakes for Vitamin a, Vitamin K, Arsenic, Boron, Chromium, Copper, Iodine, Iron, Manganese, Molybdenum, Nickel, Silicon, Vanadium, and Zinc. Washington (DC): National Academies Press (US); 2001. 7, Copper. Available from: https://www.ncbi.nlm.nih.gov/books/NBK222312/

[47] Bhattacharya PT, Misra SR, Hussain M. Nutritional aspects of essential trace elements in oral health and disease: An extensive review. Scientifica. 2016;**2016**:12-24. DOI: 10.1155/2016/54 64373

[48] Harless W, Crowell E, Abraham J. Anemia and neutropenia associated with copper deficiency of unclear etiology. American Journal of Hematology. 2006;**81**(7):546-549

[49] Trivedy CR, Warnakulasuriya KAAS, Peters TJ, Senkus R, Hazarey VK, Johnson NW. Raised tissue copper levels in oral submucous fibrosis. Journal of Oral Pathology and Medicine. 2000;**29**(6):241-248

[50] Desai VD, Kumar MVS, Bathi RJ, Gaurav I, Sharma R. Molecular analysis of trace elements in oral submucous fibrosis and future perspectives. Universal Research Journal of Dentistry. 2014;**4**(1):26-35

[51] Rajalalitha P. Molecular pathogenesis of OSMF. Journal of Oral Pathology and Medicine. 2005;**34**(6):321-328

[52] Prashanth L, Kattapagari KK, Chitturi RT, Baddam VR, Prasad LK. A

review on role of essential trace elements in health and disease. Journal of NTR University of Health Sciences. 2015;**4**:75-85

[53] Rayman MP. Selenium and human health. The Lancet. 2012;**379**(9822): 1256-1268

[54] Qamar Z, Haji Abdul Rahim ZB, Chew HP, Fatima T. Influence of trace elements on dental enamel properties: A review. Journal of the Pakistan Medical Association. 2017;**67**(1):116-120

[55] Jahangard-Rafsanjani Z, Gholami K, Hadjibabaie M, Shamshiri AR, Alimoghadam K, Sarayani A, et al. The efficacy of selenium in prevention of oral mucositis in patients undergoing hematopoietic SCT: A randomized clinical trial. Bone Marrow Transplantation. 2013;**48**(6):832-836

[56] Li Y, Widodo J, Lim S, Ooi C. Synthesis and cyto compatibility of manganese (II) and iron (III) substituted hydroxyapatite nanoparticles. Journal of Materials Science. 2012;**47**:754-763

[57] Kamberi B, Hoxha V, Kqiku L, Pertl C. The manganese content of human permanent teeth. Acta Stomatologica Croatica. 2009;**43**:83-88

[58] Broadley MR, White PJ, Hammond JP, Zelko I, Lux A. Zinc in plants. New Phytologist. 2007;**173**(4):677-702

[59] Whitney EN, Rolfes SR. Understanding Nutrition, Thomson Learning. 10th ed. Boston: Cengage Learning; 2010

[60] Franklin RB, Costello LC. Zinc as an anti-tumor agent in prostate cancer and in other cancers. Archives of Biochemistry and Biophysics. 2007;**463**:211-217

[61] Das M, Das R. Need of education and awareness towards zinc supplementation: A review. Journal of Nutrition and Metabolism. 2012;**4**(3):45-50

[62] Lynch RJ. Zinc in the mouth, its interactions with dental enamel and possible effects on caries; a review of the literature. International Dental Journal. 1984;**61**(supplement 3):46-54

[63] Henkin RI. Zinc in taste function. Biological Trace Element Research. 1984;**6**(3):263-280

[64] Das M, Das R. Need of education and awareness towards zinc supplementation: A review. International Journal of Nutrition and Metabolism. 2012;**4**(3):45-50

[65] Jayadeep A, Raveendran Pillai K, Kannan S, et al. Serum levels of copper, zinc, iron and ceruplasmin in oral leukoplakia and squamous cell carcinoma. Journal of Experimental & Clinical Cancer Research. 1997;**16**(3): 295-300

[66] Ray JG, Ghosh R, Mallick D, et al. Correlation of trace elemental profiles in blood samples of Indian patients with leukoplakia and oral submucous fibrosis. Biological Trace Element Research. 2011;**144**(1-3):295-305

[67] Mulware SJ. Trace elements and carcinogenicity: A subject in review. 3 Biotech. 2013;**3**(2):85-96

[68] Benredjem Z, Delimi R. Use of extracting agent for decadmiation of phosphate rock. Physics Procedia. 2009;**2**(3):1455-1460

[69] AlKhader AMF. The impact of phosphorus fertilizers on heavy metals content of soils and vegetables grown on selected farms in Jordan. Agrotechnology. 2015;**5**(1):1-15

[70] Arora M, Weuve J, Schwartz J, Wright RO. Association of environmental cadmium exposure with pediatric dental caries. Environmental Health Perspectives. 2008;**116**(6): 821-825

[71] Pilarczyk R, Wójcik J, Czerniak P, Sablik P, Pilarczyk B, Tomza-Marciniak A. Concentrations of toxic heavy metals and trace elements in raw milk of Simmental and Holstein-Friesian cows from organic farm. Environmental Monitoring and Assessment. 2013;**185**(10):8383-8392

[72] Mavropoulos E, Rossi AM, Costa AM, Perez CAC, Moreira JC, Saldanha M. Studies on the mechanisms of lead immobilization by hydroxyapatite. Environmental Science and Technology. 2002;**36**:1625-1629

[73] Pradeep KK, Hegde AM. Lead exposure and its relation to dentalcaries in children. The Journal of Clinical Pediatric Dentistry. 2013;**38**:71-74

[74] Abbaspour N, Hurrell R, Kelishadi R. Review on iron and its importance for human health. Journal of Research in Medical Sciences. 2014;**19**(2):164-174

[75] Gozzelino R, Arosio P. Iron homeostasis in health and disease. International Journal of Molecular Sciences. 2016;**17**(1):130

[76] Minoia C, Sabbioni E, Apostoli P, et al. Trace element reference values in tissues from inhabitants of the European community I. a study of 46 elements in urine, blood and serum of Italian subjects. Science of the Total Environment. 1990;**95**:89-105

[77] Brugnara C. Iron deficiency and erythropoiesis: New diagnostic approaches. Clinical Chemistry. 2003;**49**(10):1573-1578

[78] Labbé RF, Dewanji A. Iron assessment tests: Transferrin receptor Vis-à-Vis zinc protoporphyrin. Clinical Biochemistry. 2004;**37**(3):165-174

[79] Araya M, Pizarro F, Olivares M, Arredondo M, González M, Méndez M. Understanding copper homeostasis in humans and copper effects on health. Biological Research. 2006;**39**(1):183-187

[80] Goldman L, Ausiello D. Cecil Medicine. 23rd ed. Philadelphia, Pa, USA: Saunders Elsevier; 2007

[81] Ghadimi E, Eimar H, Marelli B, Nazhat SN, Asgharian M, Vali H, et al. Trace elements can influence the physical properties of tooth enamel. Springerplus. 2013;**2**(2):499. DOI: 10.1186/2193-1801-2-499

Chapter 3

Developmental Dental Defects and Tooth Wear: Pathological Processes Relationship

Francesco Grande and Santo Catapano

Abstract

Many conditions or pathologies can modify teeth surfaces and cause several functional and esthetic problems. Congenital dental defects and tooth wear are two of the most important reasons of dental tissue changes. Nowadays, the prevalence of tooth wear is increasing because of a high incidence of non-physiological tooth wear especially in young people. However, distinguishing dental defects originated from tooth wear or developmental dental defects is crucial to plan the most suitable treatment. Then the aim of this work is to present the different pathological conditions caused by these two etiological factors as well as the underlying biochemical mechanisms and incorrect habits related.

Keywords: tooth wear, amelogenesis imperfecta, dentinogenesis imperfecta, attrition, abrasion, erosion, abfraction

1. Introduction

Many conditions or pathologies can modify teeth surfaces and cause several functional and esthetic problems to the dental patient. They could be divided in:

- congenital defects or developmental dental defects;
- acquired dental defects.

Congenital dental defects include pathologies as amelogenesis imperfecta, dentinogenesis imperfecta and molar-incisor hypomineralization.

On the other side, dental caries, occlusal trauma and tooth wear are recognized as the most important reasons of dental tissue changes, concerning acquired dental defects. However, tooth wear has always been underrated and less considered than dental caries and trauma [1, 2]. Also congenital dental defects are little considered because of the lower prevalence in the population then dental caries although there is a clear association between some types of developmental defects and dental caries in primary dentition [3].

Regarding tooth wear, today the common opinion of dental clinicians is that the prevalence of tooth wear is increasing, because of a high incidence of non-physiological tooth wear and this is confirmed by important surveys [4, 5]. Also the prevalence of extensive wear is thought to increase, especially erosive tooth wear at young age [6].

Regarding congenital dental defects, the comprehension of genetic and environmental influences on enamel and dentine development are considered crucial for preventive actions and treatment planning of these conditions [7].

With the increased life expectancy and augmented frequency of oral hygiene procedures, problems related with tooth wear and congenital teeth defects are likely to place greater demands upon dental clinicians.

Then, in order to face that, it is important to understand the pathological mechanisms underlying developmental dental defects and dental wear and what biochemical processes and incorrect habits are involved in these conditions.

2. Congenital dental defects

Congenital dental defects are due to inherited or spontaneous genetic or epigenetic mutations that influence specialized cellular and biochemical pathways involved in dental hard tissue formation [8]. Local or systemic defects depend on where affected genes are expressed [9, 10].

However, these conditions are also caused by environmental factors such as drugs, infections, nutritional deficiencies, medical conditions or trauma [7]. Clinical importance of these defects is related to the risk of tooth decay, especially in respect of biofilm retention [11]. In addition, problems in restorative treatment because of the effectiveness of the materials and cements used for patient rehabilitation could be present.

2.1 Developmental enamel defects

Developmental enamel defects are mostly due to mutations in genes that code for enamel proteins. Generalized systemic conditions may also be present and could involve neuroectodermal mesenchyme tissues, that share common embryologic origins with enamel and dentin [12]. Otherwise, they could be induced by some pre-, peri- and postnatal factors.

Clinically, enamel abnormalities due to gene mutations are grouped under the name of amelogenesis imperfecta (AI) [7] and can be clinically divided into qualitative and quantitative defects. Qualitative defects differ from quantitative ones because they are characterized by the presence of normal amounts of enamel that is deficiently mineralized while quantitative defects are referred to enamel quantity.

Hypoplasia is a quantitative reduction of enamel formation due to disruption in ameloblast production. It can affect both the primary and permanent teeth [13]. The etiology of hypoplasia is related to insults occurring during the earliest stages of enamel development (matrix formation) [14]. It causes pits, grooves, thin or missing enamel, dental surface breaks and deficiencies.

Hypomineralization is a qualitative defect due to insults occurring in the calcification process. The resulting reduced mineralization could be recognized as soft enamel. When an altered translucency or opacity affects the entire tooth, or a localized area we can also talk of hypomaturation [12]. In case of hypomaturation and/or hypomineralization, enamel could fracture easily under loading [15] and this could result in severe tooth wear.

In the field of hypomineralization defects, a peculiar type of chronological enamel hypomineralization is the molar-incisor hypomineralization (MIH). It determines well demarcated opaque areas on the surface of permanent molars and incisors that could be colored from white to yellow or brownish, depending on the severity of the pathology [16]. In these cases, teeth often show enamel disintegration at the occlusal surfaces, post eruptive tooth structure loss and high caries susceptibility. Tooth sensitivity could also be present because of the porous prismatic enamel morphology [17]. This condition may predispose to tooth wear due to attrition between teeth and it can be aggravated in presence of other factors as abrasion and erosion. The severity of the clinical status may require extensive treatment [18–20].

Systemic factors affecting enamel development may also be distinguished in pre-, peri- and postnatal conditions in relation to the timing of the event [18] and could be caused by metabolic disturbances, drugs consumption, local infections, trauma and radiation [21, 22].

Amelogenesis defects may predispose to tooth sensitivity, plaque accumulation and increased caries risk, and in severe cases even space loss and malocclusion [23]. Also tooth wear can be associated to developmental enamel defects [7]. Infact, tooth wear could be a detrimental consequence of attrition between teeth in case of amelogenesis imperfecta and this may also cause the alteration of the normal occlusal pattern. Qualitative enamel defects may decrease the resistance of teeth both to erosion and abrasion because of the weak resistance to acid attacks and friction with foreign bodies. Furthermore, the augmented risk of dental caries and the porosity of enamel structure can enhance the process of tooth breakdown due to occlusal loading. Anterior open bite and increased calculus formation are commonly encountered in association to amelogenesis imperfecta [15] and could worsen the oral condition. Also tooth wear can be associated to developmental enamel defects.

2.2 Developmental dentin defects

Developmental dentin defects principally origin from mutations in genes coding for the proteins involved in type 1 collagen or in the extracellular matrix as well as in the mineralization processes. Defects may involve only dentine or both dentine and skeleton, if altered proteins are specific to dentine or expressed both in bone and dentine. These two types of clinical phenotype classified inherited dentine defects in the Shield's classification system [24].

Dentinogenesis imperfecta is the most common type of developmental disorder of dentine, affecting both primary and permanent teeth. It is sometimes associated with osteogenesis imperfecta [25]. When dentine and osseous defects are associated, there is a genetic fragile bone condition together with a reduced support of dentine that could show an opalescent brown discoloration. Lacking teeth support leads to easily fractures of the overlying enamel fractures as well as rapid wear and attrition of the teeth. Progressive pulp obliteration usually begins soon after eruption of the teeth and wear could arrive to the gingival level [7]. Dentine dysplasia is less common and shows normal appearing crowns with normal or short roots and pulp reduced in size. Occasionally, other abnormalities such as dental discolorations, bulbous crowns and pulp obliterations may be encountered [26].

Dentin developmental defects are highly expressed in familiar hypophosphatemia, also known as 'vitamin D-resistant rickets', an X-linked dominant inheritance condition [27]. This condition is associated with reduced resorption of phosphate in the renal tubules and characteristic rachitic bone deformities [28]. Spontaneous dental abscesses in children with no history of caries or trauma showing teeth involved in familial hypophosphatemia may occur [29]. Poorly mineralized dentine, and tubular defects extended closed to the dentino-enamel junction could predispose the pulp to exposures and infection as soon as the enamel is removed (superficial caries or attrition) [28, 30].

Because of the X-linked condition, boys are affected by the most severe dental involvement and girls the least. A wide range of spectrum manifestations has been described [26].

3. Tooth wear mechanisms

Tooth wear is defined as the progressive loss dental hard tissues from the surfaces of the teeth, caused by relative motion (friction) at the surface [1]. This type of wear includes attrition and abrasion, but also dental erosion and abfraction are nowadays included in this condition.

Tooth wear due to masticatory function is regarded as a natural phenomenon and a certain degree of tooth wear is considered unavoidable during age [31]. If the degree of destruction or the rate of loss becomes excessive, overcoming the physiological mechanisms of compensation (e.g. formation of secondary dentin), problems arise with the necessity of treatment [32]. It may cause functional and esthetic problems, dental sensitivity [1], or it could prejudice the survival of the teeth [2]. Wear could be critically pathological when it leads to poor masticatory function with concomitant reduction in quality of life and possible deterioration of systemic health [33].

The presence of developmental dental defects of enamel or dentine origin could enhance the process of tooth wear. In fact, decreased resistance in teeth with enamel and dentin abnormalities is a fact and the etiological mechanical and chemical processes of attrition, abrasion, erosion and abfraction may critically reduce the survival rate of teeth with developmental dental defects.

Then, understanding and recognizing the disruptive processes of tooth wear and if it hides possible developmental dental defects is necessary to prevent and treat several dental pathologies as worn dentition.

3.1 Attrition

Attritional is defined as the loss of tooth tissue due to friction between opposing teeth and is thus related to dental occlusion. The progressive tooth substance loss (TSL) is considered by Berry and Poole [31] a normal aging process, in which formation of secondary dentine, muscle adaptation, alveolar growth and attrition are all part of a compensation mechanism. In this view, attrition, as a normal process of changing dental morphology, should not be regarded as excessive. However, the loss of tooth tissue usually affects the dental occlusion, and it is still controversial the fact of ignoring a changing occlusion in the management of dental problems such as 'extensive' attrition or temporomandibular disorders. For these reasons and because of different assessment criteria, the exact prevalence of attrition is unclear [1, 2].

The literature on attrition does not provide clear evidence for the efficacy of particular occlusal designs in the management of attrition [34, 35]. Some cross-sectional studies [36, 37] indicate that anterior (spatial) relationships and attrition were related. As expected, anterior guidance, which is partially determined by vertical overbite and horizontal overjet, seems to reduce the risk for posterior attrition, but increases the risk for anterior attrition. Canine protection, that ensures anterior guidance, may reduce the posterior tooth substance loss but only one study tried to demonstrate it [37]. Absent posterior support did not necessarily lead to increased attrition of the remaining teeth, whereas a reduced number of teeth may lead to increased wear of the remaining teeth [38].

In dentinogenesis imperfecta, attrition is deleterious. As reported in literature, the reduced support of dentine due to genetic condition leads to easily fractures of the overlying enamel and to a progressively rapid tooth wear caused by attrition [7].

For this reason, attrition is very common in dentinogenesis imperfecta and have to be considered as one of the most important factors of tooth wear.

Attrition in patients with amelogenesis imperfecta may result in widespread exposed dentin both in primary and in permanent teeth. Deficiencies in enamel attachment to dentin and defective enamel structure take part in the process of tooth wear, that could be faster and result in dentoalveolar abnormalities because of the continuous eruption of teeth [39].

In Molar-incisor hypomineralization (MIH), tooth substance loss could be enhanced due to attrition mechanisms [40]. MIH complicated with tooth substance loss may not only compromise the esthetics and function but also endanger the pulp and longevity of the affected teeth. Tooth substance loss might be complicated by eruption of the teeth with its dentoalveolar processes which obliterate the space for any restorations [41].

Attention in these patients should also be placed when a prosthetic restoration is performed on the antagonist tooth because of the possible increased wear. The material choice is fundamental regarding mechanical properties, hardness and patient occlusion scheme, and the prosthetic restoration of the antagonist with the same material could be considered.

Attrition may be accelerated by "demastication", intended as a tooth wear process occurring during mastication of food influenced by the abrasiveness of the individual food particles [42, 43]. High levels of inorganic compounds and salts were found in snuff by Dahl et al. [44] while silica abrasive particles were also discovered in tobacco chewing by Bowles et al. [45].

Despite the possible augmented tooth substance loss because of the food particles abrasiveness, a restorative rehabilitation of the patient with developmental dental defects is important also for reestablish an appropriate food intake. In fact, the tooth wear and pain disturbances evoked by some types of food may altered patient's alimentary habits, avoiding the consumption of some important nutrients [46, 47].

Some parafunctional habits (bruxism and clenching) may contribute to attrition [1, 48]. One study concluded that excessive forceful grinding during ongoing sleep bruxism events may cause canine attrition (**Figure 1**) [49]. While the prevalence of bruxism is unclear, studies report between 5–96% of the population may be affected [1]. Its prevalence on population with developmental dental defects is not reported in literature but considering the weakness of the tooth tissues in these patients, it could be responsible of a severely worn dentition in young age [50]. Night bruxism and clenching are detrimental and a thorough dental and muscular examination has to be carried out to identify signs of bruxism and clenching in order to avoid major dental destruction. A misdiagnosis may involve future complex oral rehabilitations in order to treat patients with developmental dental defects and severe worn dentition [50].

3.2 Dental abrasion

Dental abrasion is defined as the loss of tooth substance due to friction with food and foreign body (e.g. toothbrush) and may obliterate attrition wear patterns

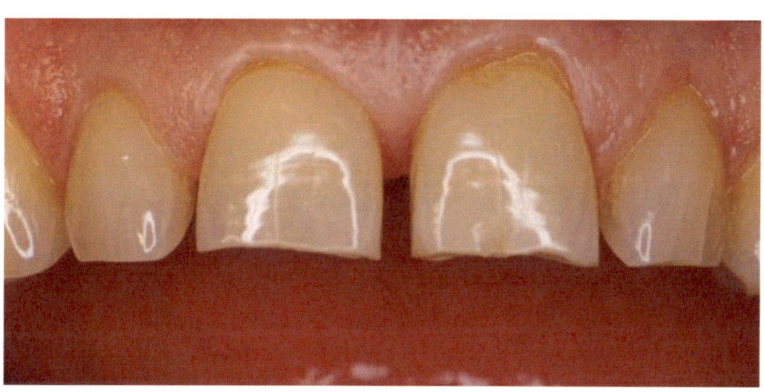

Figure 1.
A case of teeth attrition caused by bruxism.

caused by friction of opposing teeth [51]. Some types of dental abrasion may be related to habit or occupation [1, 2, 52]. Notching of incisal edges may be caused by pipe smoking, nut and seed cracking, nail biting, and hairpin biting [51, 53].

The etiology may also be deduced from the location and pattern of abrasion [52, 54]. The most common cause of dental abrasion can be found at the cervical areas and is related to toothbrushing. The technique applied, the time and frequency, the bristle design, and also the dentifrice used during toothbrushing can strongly influence this pattern [1, 48, 52]. A zealous, vigorous and repeated toothbrushing as well the use of toothbrush with not rounded tips of the bristles and abrasive dentifrice, could lead to an important dental abrasion.

In literature studies, premolars were more frequently affected with lesions varying from wedge-shaped and dish-shaped to flattened irregular and concave, with several depth and size (**Figures 2** and **3**) [55]. Data analysis revealed that vigorous toothbrushing is the major etiologic factor [56–60].

In patients with developmental dental defects, it is important to place a strong emphasis on an adequate oral home-care regimen. Education of the patient and parent guardian on an adequate tooth brushing technique and recommended oral

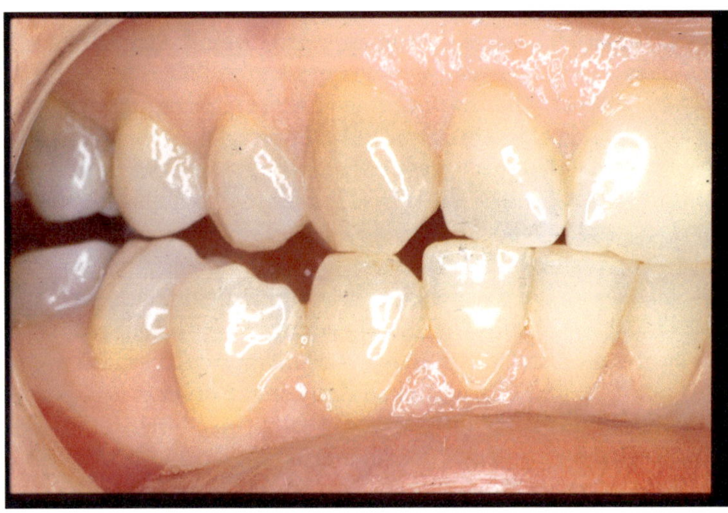

Figure 2.
Mild abrasion in canine and premolar teeth.

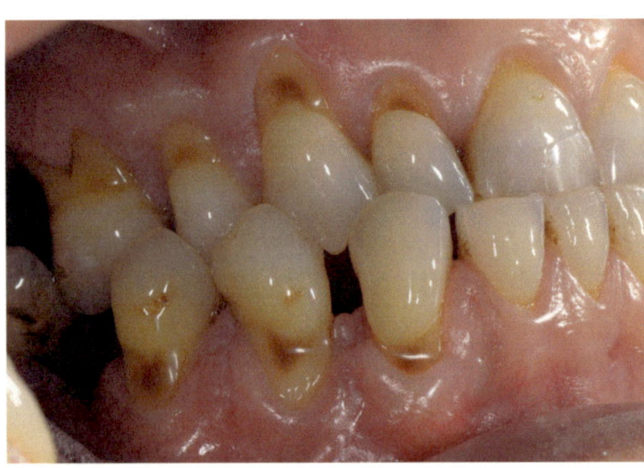

Figure 3.
Severe abrasion and abfraction lesions of the first and fourth quadrant teeth.

hygiene habits is required. Pitted enamel surfaces and roughness of teeth especially in amelogenesis imperfecta may predispose plaque accumulation and augmented susceptibility to dental caries. Oral hygiene could be poor in some patients, often because of tooth hypersensitivity and the presence of an anterior open bite associated with mouth breathing [61]. Patients have to be informed regarding their situation and instruct to maintain correct oral hygiene habitudes.

Motivation to home oral hygiene instructions is important not only for the health of hard dental tissues but also for the soft gingival tissues. Restorative procedures are usually performed in patients suffering of enamel and dentine defects. Then, teeth surfaces may retain more plaque and gingival hyperplasia can be expressed near restorations.

Dental abrasion is principally associated with horizontal brushing technique [56], but also with brush stiffness [62, 63], dentifrice abrasiveness [57, 58] and age [64, 65]. It was observed that hard bristles caused the least amount of tooth abrasion while soft bristles caused the most amount of abrasion, because of the major retention of toothpaste offered by smaller diameter filaments and denser tufts [66, 67].

Although studies show a strong association of cervical abrasions to toothbrushing, some authors affirm that dental erosion plays a great role in this tooth wear [1, 48, 63]. Experiments show that an interval of 1-hour should be considered before toothbrushing after an acid attack, in order to allow a period of remineralization necessary for improving the resistance of eroded enamel against brushing abrasion [68, 69]. Seong et al. [70] observed that enamel repair commences within 2 hours following an acidic attack and is completed 4–24 hours later. Then it could be concluded that the enamel repair process is relatively slow, exposing to high risk of tooth wear mediated by erosion/abrasion. In this context, patients with developmental dental defects and especially with enamel hypomineralization should have particular attention to avoid toothbrushing after eating acid foods and drinks. In this context, two mechanisms could accelerate tooth wear: the increased demineralization after an acid attack due to the enamel matrix hypomineralization and the reduced rate of remineralization caused by the alteration of the enamel matrix [14].

Obviously, the amount of saliva produced by each patient is one of the most important protective factors to avoid erosion of tooth structure. An appropriate evaluation of salivary rate production should be performed in this sense.

Dental hypersensitivity related to cervical abrasion and exposure of dentin to the oral environment may be possible and generally more frequent than in other populations [71].

3.3 Dental erosion

Erosion is known as the dissolution of the surface of an object by means of fluids. Dental erosion is always caused by acid dissolving hard tooth tissues [72] and has been defined as the irreversible loss of dental hard tissue caused by a chemical process not involving bacteria (**Figure 4**) [43].

A general trend of increasing tooth wear by acid erosion in particular, amongst the young people, was highlighted by several authors [73–75]. In particular, young women (15–25 years old) are often affected by psychosomatic eating disorders [76].

These phenomena often clinically overlap with other clinical pathologies such as abrasion and attrition (**Figure 5**). This could lead to a difficult differentiation, especially at the initial stages. However, as the degree of erosion increases, a more suitable differential diagnosis can be performed. It is very important to establish if dental erosion underlines any developmental dental defect that may contribute to the pathologic condition observed. And it is already fundamental to understand what type of developmental defects may affect the dentition similarly or in addition

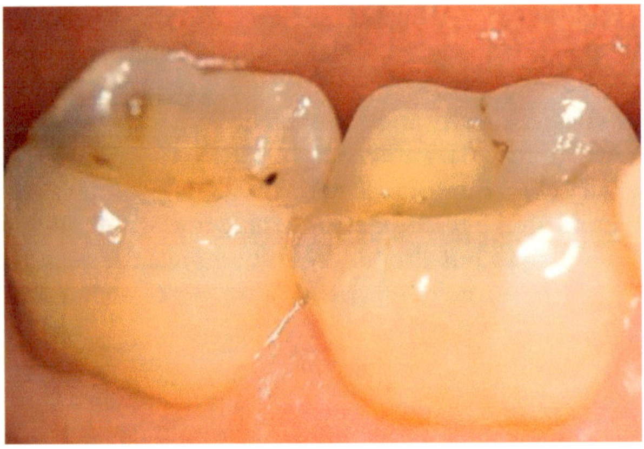

Figure 4.
Occlusal erosion of molar teeth.

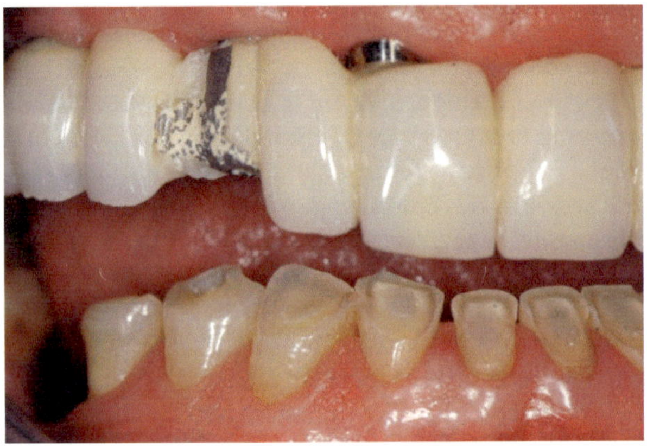

Figure 5.
Increased tooth wear of mandibular teeth cause by a combination of attrition and erosion.

to acid erosion. Sometimes, it could be difficult to distinguish if teeth with missing enamel and dental surface breaks are affected by hypoplasia, that is a quantitative reduction of enamel formation or by acids consumption. Erosion mediated by acids may also be undistinguished from enamel hypomaturation, when diffused opacities are observed. Then, the area of the opacities or structure deficiencies must be carefully observed and all the mouth have to be analyzed to understand if those defects are localized in only a part of the mouth or widespread. A correct anamnesis of the patient must also be performed regarding diet habits, gastrointestinal pathologies or drugs assumption. Dietary analysis and advice regarding erosion and sugars are fundamental to reduce further problems in teeth affected by amelogenesis imperfecta [77]. Conversely, children with AI and DI will often avoid ice cream and fridge-cold products because of the hypersensitivity and this constitute a protective factor. However, a lot of other cariogenic or acidic products may be responsible for erosion processes.

In the advanced state, the erosion can extend into dentin. The level of painful hypersensitivities as well as the esthetic or functional limitations are generally related to the extension of the erosion, although sometimes an individual component for dentin hypersensitivity may exacerbate this phenomenon. Also in this case, poorly mineralized dentine, and tubular defects in dentinogenesis imperfecta may express as extensive tooth wear, similarly to advanced case of erosion with similar hypersensitivity.

From an etiologic point of view, erosive defects can be distinguished in endogenous and exogenous. The consumption of acidic food and drugs, as well as occupational acid exposure such as wine tasters and professional swimmers, are considered extrinsic exposures [78]. Instead, intrinsic erosion is intended when gastric fluids come into contact with the oral cavity, especially in patients suffering of gastrointestinal reflux disease, eating disorders, and/or alcohol abuse [79].

Usually, a palatal and occlusal localization of the erosion defects is due to an intrinsic erosion, while an extrinsic erosion affects the labial surfaces of the anterior teeth [80]. Both types of erosion produce deleterious effects on dental elements, with a pattern of destruction dependent on the erosivity of the erosion-causing solution (pH, buffer capacity, and mineral concentration), and also on the frequency and type of acid exposure. However, as gastric fluid is evaluated as 1 in the pH scale and is provided with a high amount of free acid, its erosive potential is higher than that of extrinsic acids [81]. Moreover, patients with eating disorders often show xerostomia because of the lower salivary flow rate caused by the general dehydration or by the antidepressant drugs, which could further increase the risk of developing erosive lesions.

3.4 Abfraction

Abfraction or Non Carious Cervical Lesions (NCCL) have been used to describe wedge shaped cervical lesions as a wear defect [82]. It is recognized as the loss of cervical tooth tissues induced by mechanical loading which led to enamel and dentin flexure and failure [83]. Some biomechanical analyses show that the most important area of stress concentration is located at the cervical areas of the teeth in response to overloading, that leads to initiation of a cervical lesion [84, 85].

Another study, using FEM, suggested that oblique loading on the tooth stretches the enamel surface near the cemento-enamel junction causing plastic deformation at the cervical area [86]. It was seen that lateral forces produce compressive stresses on the side toward which the tooth bends and the tensile stresses are on the other side. These stresses create microfractures at the cervical region which propagate perpendicularly to the long axis of the tooth, leading to a localized defect around the CEJ [87]. The tensile forces could disrupt the hydroxyapatite (HA) crystals of the enamel structure, allowing saliva and other small molecules to penetrate between the prisms and prevent re-establishment of the interprismatic bonds on release of the stress (**Figure 6**). Ultimately, when the enamel breaks away at the cervical margin and exposes the dentin, the process continues in this way and may accelerate because of the structure of the dentin [82].

Cervical lesions depend on type and severity of the etiologic factor, and not all these lesions require restorations. They appear primarily at the cervical region of the dentition and are typically wedge-shaped, with sharp internal and external line angles [55].

Treatment planning of non carious cervical lesions is based on the reduction of stress concentration in order to strengthen the tooth, the prevention of dentin hypersensitivity with major pulp protection and the modification of oral hygiene habits, improving also the esthetics [82]. Composites and glass ionomer restorations can be adopted if lesions are not too much extended. On the other hand, metal crowns can be used where the masticatory load is higher. In order to treat hypersensitivity, dentin bonding agents, fluoride varnishes and other desensitizing agents may be useful. Gnatologic devices also can be fabricated to protect teeth during night, however changing of dietary and oral habits is mandatory [88, 89].

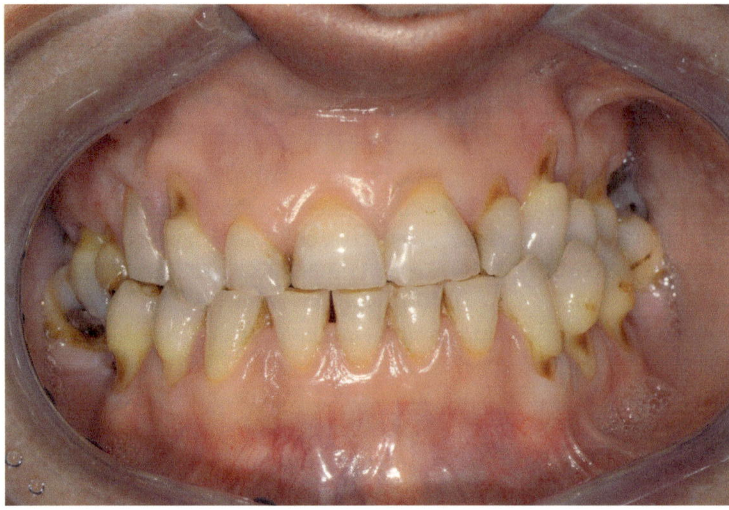

Figure 6.
Abfraction lesions associated with moderate tooth wear.

4. Diagnosis and management of patients with developmental dental defects and tooth wear

Tooth wear is multifactorial in origin [51]. The major factors responsible for tooth wear should be identified starting from a correct and thorough anamnesis of the patient in order to establish a predictable treatment plan. Several signs may result useful in the differential diagnosis process and the appearance of worn tooth surfaces resulting from the various types of wear differ. In order to make a correct diagnosis of the etiology of tooth wear it is fundamental not only to observe the wear pattern but also to investigate if any erosive or abrasive factor is present in the anamnesis. However, if a clear etiological factor is not find, the observed tooth wear may be due to the mechanical type. However, identification and recognition of developmental dental defects is of extreme importance (**Table 1**) [23, 94]. In fact, early diagnosis and preventive care are essential for the successful treatment of developmental dental defects. Children with a family history of amelogenesis or dentinogenesis imperfecta, or medical syndromes commonly associated with them such as prematurity of birth or hypophosphatemia should be assessed for developmental dental defects as soon as the teeth erupt. Defects in primary teeth may possibly indicate a risk also for permanent dentition [7].

For children with developmental dental defects, a preventive program should be instituted immediately after diagnosis. Neutral sodium fluoride gels or varnishes professional applications every 3/6 months, in addition with calcium and phosphate rich agents (casein phosphopeptide-amorphous calcium phosphate, CPP-ACP) are recommended to reduce caries risk and developmental opacities in teeth with enamel hypoplasia [95]. Because of the structural weakness of the teeth with developmental dental defects, other important recommendations are the same as erosive protection advices such as reduced consumption of acidic food, diet and soft drinks, control of eventual psychosomatic disorders, because of the possibility of frequent vomiting [90]. It is also important to consider that the risk of erosive lesions is increased when acid or soft drinks are assumed by children from a feeding bottle at bed- or nap-time, because of the lower salivary flow rate during sleep [96]. Furthermore, several drinking habits (sips drinking, use of a straw in direct contact with teeth, and intensive rinsing) cause a prolonged pH drop in the oral

	Etiology	Clinical signs	Preventive and possible therapeutic options
Attrition	Friction between opposing teeth [72]	Occlusal tooth wear	Teeth prosthetic or conservative restorations [1, 2]
Erosion	Contact between acid substances and teeth [43]	Vestibular, palatal and/or occlusal tooth substance loss	Avoid acid foods and drinks consumption [90, 91]
Abrasion	Friction between teeth and foreign body [72]	Cervical vestibular tooth substance loss	Avoid horizontal toothbrushing technique and dental abrasive habits [48, 52]
Enamel hypoplasia	Quantitative reduction of enamel formation [12]	Thin enamel area with surface pitting or vertical grooving on several teeth	Microabrasion and restorative or prosthetic treatment [12, 92]
Enamel hypomineralization	Reduced enamel mineralization [40, 93]	Soft and/or discolored enamel	Fluoride applications, restorative and/or prosthetic treatment [16, 17]
Dentinogenesis imperfecta	Alterations in collagen proteins [47]	Tooth discoloration, enamel fractures, pulp obliteration	Prophylactic coverage with stainless steel crowns, Fluoride applications [7]

Table 1.
Summary table of the etiology, clinical signs and preventive and therapeutic options of developmental dental defects and tooth wear conditions. Clinicians must consider possible associations between these two pathological entities.

cavity compared to a short consumption [97]. Then, patients should restrict the consumption of acidic food and drinks only to main meals. Acidic beverages should be consumed cool and as fast as possible in order to reduce their erosivity. Some foods as yogurts that have high concentrations of calcium and phosphate, result non-erosive despite their low pH [91].

When tooth wear is already present, the treatment planning in children with extensive enamel defects due to may involve complex restorations, orthodontics, exodontia and prosthodontics [77].

Normally, without any developmental dental defects, the treatment planning depends on the severity of tooth wear. The amount of tooth wear necessary for intervention is not clear from the scientific literature, even if with the Smith and Knight index [98], the threshold to start restorative treatment is set once dentine was involved. A recent paper summarizes when it is recommended a restorative treatment [99]. Another paper indicates several techniques and treatment strategies for tooth wear, clearly distinguishing between pathological and physiological tooth wear; it is also highlighted that dentist has to detect the speed and severity of tooth wear process in order to decide when intervening [100]. However, difficulties in detecting a pathological dental loss at early stages differently from physiological loss, is challenging for the dentist. A complicating factor is also that tooth wear may be cyclical and can be inactive in the majority of the patients, despite obvious wear facets in their dentitions [101].

However, in developmental dental defects, because the structural weakness of the hard tissues leads to its readily deterioration under masticatory stresses and both amelogenesis and dentinogenesis imperfecta are associated with rapid toothwear and crown fractures, protection from toothwear is recommended soon after eruption [102]. Ideally, restorative stabilization of the dentition should be completed before excessive wear and loss of vertical dimension occur [103]. Guidelines for the treatment of developmental dental anomalies have been established by AAPD (American Academy of Pediatric Dentistry) [104]. For developmental enamel defects, treatment should begin as soon as possible according to patient compliance in office dental care. Early identification and preventive interventions are critical for infants and children with enamel defects due to amelogenesis imperfecta in order to avoid the negative social and functional consequences of the disorder. The appearance, quality, and amount of affected enamel and dentin will dictate the type of restorations necessary to achieve esthetic, masticatory, and functional health. Depending on the severity of enamel defects and tooth wear, treatment can range from bleaching and/or microabrasion [92] to composite resin, porcelain veneers [105] or full coverage restorations with crowns placement [39].

Treatment of dentinogenesis imperfecta frequently includes preventing severe attrition associated with enamel loss and rapid wear of the poorly mineralized dentin, rehabilitating dentitions that have undergone severe wear, optimizing esthetics, and preventing caries and periodontal disease [104].

Stainless steel crowns are a highly durable restoration choice for the prophylactic coverage of teeth affect by developmental dental defects. In teeth with dentine defects, they reduce the risk of pulp exposure and infection, especially in some types of dentine defects (hypophosphatemia) [28]. Fluoride applications and desensitizing agents may also diminish tooth sensitivity [106]. In teeth affected by enamel hypoplasia both primary and permanent molars show a reduction in tooth sensitivity and in cusp fractures after prosthetic rehabilitation with stainless teel crowns. This also helps to maintain space and crown height, important also for orthodontic issues. The crowns are best inserted using a conservative technique, originally proposed by Seow, that involves a minimal removal of tooth structure in order to protect teeth with large pulps and dentin defects [28, 107]. In adulthood, the stainless steel crowns may be replaced with gold or porcelain crowns to provide long term protection of the teeth.

It should also be considered that marginal leakage around restorations and recurrent caries with eventual pulp involvement may be determined from the enamel deterioration [108, 109]. Materials as resin modified glass-ionomer cements and polyacid modified composites should be used for restoring teeth affected by enamel defects in order to take advantage of the optimal bonding of these material with both dentine and enamel [110]. However, despite their esthetic value, composite resins have low adhesion to poorly mineralized enamel. Then, it is important to consider the amount of tooth wear in order to proceed with conservative or prosthetic rehabilitation.

In cases with significant loss of vertical dimension because of tooth wear, the reestablishment of a more normal vertical dimension is crucial for a correct function, mastication and esthetics. Cases showing severe loss of coronal tooth structure and vertical dimension have to be considered candidates for overdenture therapy. Overlay dentures placed on teeth that are covered with fluoride-releasing glass ionomer cement have also been used with success [111].

Conflict of interest

The authors declare no conflict of interest.

Author details

Francesco Grande* and Santo Catapano
Dental School, Dental Clinic, University of Ferrara, Ferrara, Italy

*Address all correspondence to: francesco.grande90@gmail.com

References

[1] Bishop K, Kelleher M, Briggs P, Joshi R. Wear now? An update on the etiology of tooth wear. Quintessence Int. 1997 May;28(5):305-313.

[2] Kelleher M, Bishop K. Tooth surface loss: An overview. Br Dent J. 1999 Jan 23;186(2):61-66.

[3] Costa FS, Silveira ER, Pinto GS, Nascimento GG, Thomson WM, Demarco FF. Developmental defects of enamel and dental caries in the primary dentition: A systematic review and meta-analysis. J Dent. 2017 May;60:1-7.

[4] White DA, Tsakos G, Pitts NB, Fuller E, Douglas GVA, Murray JJ, et al. Adult dental health survey 2009: Common oral health conditions and their impact on the population. Br Dent J. 2012 Dec;213(11):567-572.

[5] Salas MMS, Nascimento GG, Huysmans MC, Demarco FF. Estimated prevalence of erosive tooth wear in permanent teeth of children and adolescents: An epidemiological systematic review and meta-regression analysis. J Dent. 2015 Jan;43(1):42-50.

[6] Arnadottir IB, Holbrook WP, Eggertsson H, Gudmundsdottir H, Jonsson SH, Gudlaugsson JO, et al. Prevalence of dental erosion in children: A national survey. Community Dent Oral Epidemiol. 2010 Dec;38(6): 521-526.

[7] Seow W. Developmental defects of enamel and dentine: Challenges for basic science research and clinical management. Aust Dent J. 2014 Jun;59:143-154.

[8] Brook AH. Multilevel complex interactions between genetic, epigenetic and environmental factors in the aetiology of anomalies of dental development. Arch Oral Biol. 2009 Dec;54 Suppl 1:S3-17.

[9] Wright JT, Hart TC, Hart PS, Simmons D, Suggs C, Daley B, et al. Human and mouse enamel phenotypes resulting from mutation or altered expression of AMEL, ENAM, MMP20 and KLK4. Cells Tissues Organs. 2009;189(1-4):224-229.

[10] Forlino A, Cabral WA, Barnes AM, Marini JC. New perspectives on osteogenesis imperfecta. Nat Rev Endocrinol. 2011 Jun 14;7(9):540-557.

[11] Li Y, Navia JM, Caufield PW. Colonization by mutans streptococci in the mouths of 3- and 4-year-old Chinese children with or without enamel hypoplasia. Archives of Oral Biology. 1994 Dec;39(12):1057-1062.

[12] Pascoe L, Seow WK. Enamel hypoplasia and dental caries in Australian aboriginal children: Prevalence and correlation between the two diseases. Pediatr Dent. 1994 Jun;16(3):193-199.

[13] Witkop CJ. Amelogenesis imperfecta, dentinogenesis imperfecta and dentin dysplasia revisited: Problems in classification. J Oral Pathol. 1988 Nov;17(9-10):547-553.

[14] Wright JT. The molecular etiologies and associated phenotypes of amelogenesis imperfecta. Am J Med Genet A. 2006 Dec 1;140(23):2547-2555.

[15] Seow WK. Clinical diagnosis and management strategies of amelogenesis imperfectavariants. Pediatr Dent. 1993 Dec;15(6):384-393.

[16] Weerheijm KL, Jälevik B, Alaluusua S. Molar-incisor hypomineralisation. Caries Res. 2001 Oct;35(5):390-391.

[17] Jälevik B, Klingberg GA. Dental treatment, dental fear and behaviour management problems in children with severe enamel hypomineralization of

their permanent first molars. Int J Paediatr Dent. 2002 Jan;12(1):24-32.

[18] Ford D, Seow WK, Kazoullis S, Holcombe T, Newman B. A controlled study of risk factors for enamel hypoplasia in the permanent dentition. Pediatr Dent. 2009 Oct;31(5):382-388.

[19] Whatling R, Fearne JM. Molar incisor hypomineralization: A study of aetiological factors in a group of UK children. Int J Paediatr Dent. 2008 May;18(3):155-162.

[20] Rugg-Gunn AJ, Al-Mohammadi SM, Butler TJ. Malnutrition and developmental defects of enamel in 2- to 6-year-old Saudi boys. Caries Res. 1998;32(3):181-192.

[21] Pöyhönen H, Nurmi M, Peltola V, Alaluusua S, Ruuskanen O, Lähdesmäki T. Dental staining after doxycycline use in children. J Antimicrob Chemother. 2017 Oct 1;72(10):2887-2890.

[22] Bardellini E, Amadori F, Pasini S, Majorana A. Dental anomalies in permanent teeth after trauma in primary dentition. J Clin Pediatr Dent. 2017;41(1):5-9.

[23] Seow WK, Humphrys C, Tudehope DI. Increased prevalence of developmental dental defects in low birth-weight, prematurely born children: A controlled study. Pediatr Dent. 1987 Sep;9(3):221-225.

[24] Shields ED, Bixler D, el-Kafrawy AM. A proposed classification for heritable human dentine defects with a description of a new entity. Arch Oral Biol. 1973 Apr;18(4):543-553.

[25] Biria M, Abbas FM, Mozaffar S, Ahmadi R. Dentinogenesis imperfecta associated with osteogenesis imperfecta. Dent Res J (Isfahan). 2012 Jul;9(4):489-494.

[26] Seow WK, Shusterman S. Spectrum of dentin dysplasia in a family: Case report and literature review. Pediatr Dent. 1994 Dec;16(6):437-442.

[27] Carpenter TO. The expanding family of hypophosphatemic syndromes. J Bone Miner Metab. 2012 Jan;30(1):1-9.

[28] Seow WK, Latham SC. The spectrum of dental manifestations in vitamin D-resistant rickets: Implications for management. Pediatr Dent. 1986 Sep;8(3):245-250.

[29] Seow WK. Diagnosis and management of unusual dental abscesses in children. Aust Dent J. 2003 Sep;48(3):156-168.

[30] Seow WK, Romaniuk K, Sclavos S. Micromorphologic features of dentin in vitamin D-resistant rickets: Correlation with clinical grading of severity. Pediatr Dent. 1989 Sep;11(3):203-208.

[31] Berry DC, Poole DF. Attrition: Possible mechanisms of compensation. J Oral Rehabil. 1976 Jul;3(3):201-206.

[32] Milosevic A. Toothwear: Management. Dent Update. 1998 Mar;25(2):50-55.

[33] DeLong R. Intra-oral restorative materials wear: Rethinking the current approaches: How to measure wear. Dent Mater. 2006 Aug;22(8):702-711.

[34] Johansson A, Fareed K, Omar R. Lateral and protrusive contact schemes and occlusal wear: A correlational study in a young adult Saudi population. J Prosthet Dent. 1994 Feb;71(2):159-164.

[35] Abdullah A, Sherfudhin H, Omar R, Johansson A. Prevalence of occlusal tooth wear and its relationship to lateral and protrusive contact schemes in a young adult Indian population. Acta Odontol Scand. 1994 Aug;52(4):191-197.

[36] Bauer W, van den Hoven F, Diedrich P. Wear in the upper and lower incisors in relation to incisal and condylar guidance. J Orofac Orthop. 1997;58(6):306-319.

[37] Seligman DA, Pullinger AG. The degree to which dental attrition in modern society is a function of age and of canine contact. J Orofac Pain. 1995;9(3):266-275.

[38] van 't Spijker A, Kreulen CM, Creugers NHJ. Attrition, occlusion, (dys)function, and intervention: a systematic review. Clin Oral Implants Res. 2007 Jun;18 Suppl 3:117-26.

[39] Yip HK, Smales RJ. Oral rehabilitation of young adults with amelogenesis imperfecta. Int J Prosthodont. 2003 Aug;16(4):345-349.

[40] Lam WYH, Ho EHT, Pow EHN. Rehabilitation of molar-incisor hypomineralization (MIH) complicated with localized tooth surface loss: A case report. Quintessence Int. 2014 May;45(5):377-379.

[41] Poyser NJ, Porter RWJ, Briggs PFA, Chana HS, Kelleher MGD. The Dahl concept: Past, present and future. Br Dent J. 2005 Jun 11;198(11):669-676; quiz 720.

[42] Moss SJ. Dental erosion. Int Dent J. 1998 Dec;48(6):529-539.

[43] Imfeld T. Dental erosion. Definition, classification and links. Eur J Oral Sci. 1996 Apr;104(2 (Pt 2)):151-5.

[44] Dahl BL, Stølen SO, Oilo G. Abrasives in snuff? Acta Odontol Scand. 1989 Aug;47(4):239-243.

[45] Bowles WH, Wilkinson MR, Wagner MJ, Woody RD. Abrasive particles in tobacco products: A possible factor in dental attrition. J Am Dent Assoc. 1995 Mar;126(3):327-331; quiz 348.

[46] Sabandal MMI, Dammaschke T, Schäfer E. Restorative treatment in a case of amelogenesis imperfecta and 9-year follow-up: A case report. Head Face Med. 2020 Nov 19;16(1):28.

[47] Abukabbos H, Al-Sineedi F. Clinical manifestations and dental management of dentinogenesis imperfecta associated with osteogenesis imperfecta: Case report. Saudi Dent J. 2013 Oct;25(4):159-165.

[48] Bartlett D, Phillips K, Smith B. a difference in perspective--the north American and European interpretations of tooth wear. Int J Prosthodont. 1999 Oct;12(5):401-408.

[49] Okura K, Shigemoto S, Suzuki Y, Noguchi N, Omoto K, Abe S, et al. Mandibular movement during sleep bruxism associated with current tooth attrition. Journal of Prosthodontic Research. 2017 Jan;61(1):87-95.

[50] Tang Y, Cao T, Zhang L, Bao G, Kang H. Restoration of the dentition in a patient with a history of bruxism and amelogenesis imperfecta: A clinical report. Clin Case Rep. 2021 Feb;9(2):898-905.

[51] Litonjua LA, Andreana S, Bush PJ, Cohen RE. Tooth wear: Attrition, erosion, and abrasion. Quintessence Int. 2003 Jun;34(6):435-446.

[52] Hattab FN, Yassin OM. Etiology and diagnosis of tooth wear: A literature review and presentation of selected cases. Int J Prosthodont. 2000 Apr;13(2):101-107.

[53] Amin W, Kassab A, Salim N. Incisal Edge Abrasion Caused By An Unusual Eating Habit. The Internet Journal of Dental Science [Internet]. 2007;6(1). Available from: https://print.ispub.com/api/0/ispub-article/13040

[54] Johnson GK, Sivers JE. Attrition, abrasion and erosion: Diagnosis and

therapy. Clin Prev Dent. 1987 Oct;9(5):12-16.

[55] Nascimento MM, Dilbone DA, Pereira PN, Duarte WR, Geraldeli S, Delgado AJ. Abfraction lesions: Etiology, diagnosis, and treatment options. Clin Cosmet Investig Dent. 2016;8:79-87.

[56] Bergström J, Lavstedt S. An epidemiologic approach to toothbrushing and dental abrasion. Community Dent Oral Epidemiol. 1979 Feb;7(1):57-64.

[57] Cohen RB. Toothpaste abrasion. J Am Dent Assoc. 2004 Nov;135(11):1520, 1522; author reply 1522.

[58] Presswood RG, Townsend G, Kaidonis J. The use of toothpaste precipitates wear patterns. J Prosthet Dent. 2013 Dec;110(6):544.

[59] Linn H. Toothpaste abuse? J Am Dent Assoc. 2005 Jan;136(1):22, 24; author reply 24, 26.

[60] Hand JS, Hunt RJ, Reinhardt JW. The prevalence and treatment implications of cervical abrasion in the elderly. Gerodontics. 1986 Oct;2(5):167-170.

[61] Rowley R, Hill FJ, Winter GB. An investigation of the association between anterior open-bite and amelogenesis imperfecta. Am J Orthod. 1982 Mar;81(3):229-235.

[62] Björn H, Lindhe J. Abrasion of dentine by toothbrush and dentifrice. A methodological study. Odontol Revy. 1966;17(1):17-27.

[63] Sangnes G. Traumatization of teeth and gingiva related to habitual tooth cleaning procedures. J Clin Periodontol. 1976 May;3(2):94-103.

[64] Splieth CH, Tachou A. Epidemiology of dentin hypersensitivity. Clin Oral Investig. 2013 Mar;17 Suppl 1:S3-S8.

[65] Brady JM, Woody RD. Scanning microscopy of cervical erosion. J Am Dent Assoc. 1977 Apr;94(4):726-729.

[66] Dyer D, Addy M, Newcombe RG. Studies in vitro of abrasion by different manual toothbrush heads and a standard toothpaste. J Clin Periodontol. 2000 Feb;27(2):99-103.

[67] Davis WB, Winter PJ. Measurement in vitro of enamel abrasion by dentifrice. J Dent Res. 1976 Dec;55(6):970-975.

[68] Attin T, Buchalla W, Gollner M, Hellwig E. Use of variable remineralization periods to improve the abrasion resistance of previously eroded enamel. Caries Res. 2000 Feb;34(1):48-52.

[69] Jaeggi T, Lussi A. Toothbrush abrasion of erosively altered enamel after intraoral exposure to saliva: An in situ study. Caries Res. 1999 Dec;33(6):455-461.

[70] Seong J, Virani A, Parkinson C, Claydon N, Hellin N, Newcombe RG, et al. Clinical enamel surface changes following an intra-oral acidic challenge. J Dent. 2015 Aug;43(8):1013-1020.

[71] West NX, Lussi A, Seong J, Hellwig E. Dentin hypersensitivity: Pain mechanisms and aetiology of exposed cervical dentin. Clin Oral Investig. 2013 Mar;17 Suppl 1:S9-19.

[72] Grippo JO, Simring M, Schreiner S. Attrition, abrasion, corrosion and abfraction revisited: A new perspective on tooth surface lesions. J Am Dent Assoc. 2004 Aug;135(8):1109-1118; quiz 1163-5.

[73] Jaeggi T, Lussi A. Prevalence, incidence and distribution of erosion. Monogr Oral Sci. 2014;25:55-73.

[74] Marthaler TM. Changes in dental caries 1953-2003. Caries Res. 2004 Jun;38(3):173-181.

[75] Nunn JH, Gordon PH, Morris AJ, Pine CM, Walker A. Dental erosion—Changing prevalence? A review of British national childrens' surveys. Int J Paediatr Dent. 2003 Mar;13(2):98-105.

[76] Imfeld C, Imfeld T. [Eating disorders (II)--dental aspects]. Schweiz Monatsschr Zahnmed. 2005;115(12):1163-1171.

[77] McDonald S, Arkutu N, Malik K, Gadhia K, McKaig S. Managing the paediatric patient with amelogenesis imperfecta. Br Dent J. 2012 May 11;212(9):425-428.

[78] Rao KA, Thomas S, Kumar JK, Narayan V. Prevalence of dentinal hypersensitivity and dental Erosion among competitive swimmers, Kerala, India. Indian J Community Med. 2019 Dec;44(4):390-393.

[79] Bartlett D. Intrinsic causes of erosion. Monogr Oral Sci. 2006;20:119-139.

[80] Kanzow P, Wegehaupt FJ, Attin T, Wiegand A. Etiology and pathogenesis of dental erosion. Quintessence Int. 2016 Apr;47(4):275-278.

[81] Uhlen M-M, Tveit AB, Stenhagen KR, Mulic A. Self-induced vomiting and dental erosion--a clinical study. BMC Oral Health. 2014 Jul 29;14:92.

[82] Bartlett DW, Shah P. A critical review of non-carious cervical (wear) lesions and the role of abfraction, erosion, and abrasion. J Dent Res. 2006 Apr;85(4):306-312.

[83] Sarode GS, Sarode SC. Abfraction: A review. J Oral Maxillofac Pathol. 2013 May;17(2):222-227.

[84] Litonjua LA, Andreana S, Patra AK, Cohen RE. An assessment of stress analyses in the theory of abfraction. Biomed Mater Eng. 2004;14(3):311-321.

[85] Dejak B, Mlotkowski A, Romanowicz M. Finite element analysis of mechanism of cervical lesion formation in simulated molars during mastication and parafunction. J Prosthet Dent. 2005 Dec;94(6):520-529.

[86] Tanaka M, Naito T, Yokota M, Kohno M. Finite element analysis of the possible mechanism of cervical lesion formation by occlusal force. J Oral Rehabil. 2003 Jan;30(1):60-67.

[87] Romeed SA, Malik R, Dunne SM. Stress analysis of occlusal forces in canine teeth and their role in the development of non-carious cervical lesions: Abfraction. Int J Dent. 2012;2012:234845.

[88] Coleman TA, Grippo JO, Kinderknecht KE. Cervical dentin hypersensitivity. Part II: Associations with abfractive lesions. Quintessence Int. 2000 Aug;31(7):466-473.

[89] Hayes M, Brady P, Burke FM, Allen PF. Failure rates of class V restorations in the management of root caries in adults—A systematic review. Gerodontology. 2016 Sep;33(3):299-307.

[90] Hermont AP, Oliveira PAD, Martins CC, Paiva SM, Pordeus IA, Auad SM. Tooth erosion and eating disorders: A systematic review and meta-analysis. PLoS One. 2014;9(11):e111123.

[91] Barbour ME, Lussi A. Erosion in relation to nutrition and the environment. Monogr Oral Sci. 2014;25:143-154.

[92] Ashkenazi M, Sarnat H. Microabrasion of teeth with discoloration resembling hypomaturation enamel defects: Four-year follow up. J Clin Pediatr Dent. 2000;25(1):29-34.

[93] Ghanim A, Mariño R, Morgan M, Bailey D, Manton D. An in vivo investigation of salivary properties,

enamel hypomineralisation, and carious lesion severity in a group of Iraqi schoolchildren. Int J Paediatr Dent. 2013 Jan;23(1):2-12.

[94] Arrow P. Prevalence of developmental enamel defects of the first permanent molars among school children in Western Australia. Aust Dent J. 2008 Sep;53(3):250-259.

[95] Cochrane NJ, Reynolds EC. Calcium phosphopeptides—Mechanisms of action and evidence for clinical efficacy. Adv Dent Res. 2012 Sep;24(2):41-47.

[96] Al-Malik MI, Holt RD, Bedi R. The relationship between erosion, caries and rampant caries and dietary habits in preschool children in Saudi Arabia. Int J Paediatr Dent. 2001 Nov;11(6):430-439.

[97] Johansson A-K, Lingström P, Birkhed D. Comparison of factors potentially related to the occurrence of dental erosion in high- and low-erosion groups. Eur J Oral Sci. 2002 Jun;110(3):204-211.

[98] Smith BG, Knight JK. An index for measuring the wear of teeth. Br Dent J. 1984 Jun 23;156(12):435-438.

[99] Loomans B, Opdam N, Attin T, Bartlett D, Edelhoff D, Frankenberger R, et al. Severe tooth Wear: European consensus statement on management guidelines. J Adhes Dent. 2017;19(2):111-119.

[100] Loomans B, Opdam N. A guide to managing tooth wear: the Radboud philosophy. Br Dent J. 2018 09;224(5):348-56.

[101] Rodriguez JM, Austin RS, Bartlett DW. In vivo measurements of tooth wear over 12 months. Caries Res. 2012;46(1):9-15.

[102] Seow WK, Taji S. Diagnosis and management of toothwear in children. In: Khan F, Young WG, eds. Toothwear: The ABC of the Worn Dentition. Chichester, West Sussex, UK: Wiley-Blackwell, 2011:16-33.

[103] Sapir S, Shapira J. Dentinogenesis imperfecta: An early treatment strategy. Pediatr Dent. 2001 Jun;23(3):232-237.

[104] American Academy of Pediatric Dentistry. Guideline on dental management of heritable dental developmental anomalies. Pediatr Dent. 2013 Oct;35(5):E179-E184.

[105] Sengun A, Ozer F. Restoring function and esthetics in a patient with amelogenesis imperfecta: A case report. Quintessence Int. 2002 Mar;33(3):199-204.

[106] Sapir S, Shapira J. Clinical solutions for developmental defects of enamel and dentin in children. Pediatr Dent. 2007 Aug;29(4):330-336.

[107] Kwok-Tung L, King NM. The restorative management of amelogenesis imperfecta in the mixed dentition. J Clin Pediatr Dent. 2006;31(2):130-135.

[108] Mejàre I, Bergman E, Grindefjord M. Hypomineralized molars and incisors of unknown origin: Treatment outcome at age 18 years. Int J Paediatr Dent. 2005 Jan;15(1):20-28.

[109] Kotsanos N, Kaklamanos EG, Arapostathis K. Treatment management of first permanent molars in children with molar-incisor Hypomineralisation. Eur J Paediatr Dent. 2005 Dec;6(4):179-184.

[110] Chadwick BL, Evans DJP. Restoration of class II cavities in primary molar teeth with conventional and resin modified glass ionomer cements: A systematic review of the literature. Eur Arch Paediatr Dent. 2007 Mar;8(1):14-21.

[111] Neville BW, Damm DD, Allen CM, Bouquot JE. Abnormalities of teeth. In: Oral & Maxillofacial Pathology. 2nd ed. Philadelphia, Pa: WB Saunders Company; 2002: 89-99.

Section 2

Genetic Components of Developmental Dental Defects

Chapter 4

Failure of Tooth Development: Prevalence, Genetic Causes and Clinical Features

Emilia Severin, George Gabriel Moldoveanu and Andreea Moldoveanu

Abstract

In dental practice may be encountered a wide variability in the clinical dental phenotype of tooth number. Failure of tooth development at the bud stage causes tooth agenesis and reduction in tooth number in the dental arch which involves various complications. Tooth agenesis is one of the most common developmental anomalies of human permanent dentition and tends to run in families, may aggregate within families, suggesting a genetic cause. Tooth agenesis can occur in association with a variety of craniofacial syndromes, but it is also found as an isolated trait (familial or sporadic). Other tooth anomalies, such as tooth shape and size, delayed eruption of teeth, malposition, short roots or taurodontism, have been noted in association with non-syndromic tooth agenesis as well. Both the deciduous and permanent dentitions may be affected by missing teeth. Variations in the number of missing teeth can be determined by a mutation in one gene, by mutations in multiple genes, induced by local or systemically acting environmental factor, caused by a combination of gene mutations and environmental factors acting together, or by damage to chromosomes. As the number of missing teeth increases, so does the severity of clinical consequences and the impact on oral health–related quality of life.

Keywords: abnormalities in the tooth number, tooth agenesis, missing teeth, hypodontia, oligodontia

1. Introduction

The craniofacial growth and its harmonization with the dental apparatus take place according to a genetic program that acts in a coordinated manner, in both embryo foetal and postnatal stages. In addition to the structural pattern of development, the genetic program also ensures the control of each stage of ontogenesis, both in space and time, which eliminates the risk of developmental errors. During odontogenesis intricate genetic, molecular and cellular regulations establish accurate tooth number and precise location, size, morphology, and composition of each tooth.

However, deviations from usual structure, or function are possible. Any deviation, qualitative and/or quantitative, from usual pattern of development may be called developmental abnormality or anomaly. Developmental anomalies are also known as congenital anomalies or birth defects. Congenital anomalies are defined by the World Health Organization (WHO)"as structural or functional anomalies". They can occur during antenatal life and can be detected"prenatally, at birth, or later in infancy" [1].

Development failure of one or more teeth is a result of specific disturbances (failure in the initiation of tooth formation, reduced odontogenic potential of the dental lamina, or premature arrest of tooth development) during the early stages (tooth initiation or morphogenesis stage) of odontogenesis affecting reciprocal interactions between the dental epithelium and mesenchyme and leading to absence of tooth germ [2]. Therefore, the usual number of deciduous and permanent dentitions, in both jaws, decrease and the condition is known as tooth agenesis. Family, twin, adoption and tooth development at molecular levels studies provide evidence-based interpretation of genetics as the predominant factors in the etiology of tooth agenesis. Frequently association of tooth agenesis with inherited monogenic syndromes supports the role of genetics in the etiology of missing teeth.

Absence of tooth developmental has direct clinical implications causing physical appearance, emotional, and functional impact on the affected individual. Most affected individuals lack only one or two permanent teeth, but patients who experience agenesis of more teeth are frequently encountered in dental practice as well. Severe forms of missing teeth lead to greater oral impairments. The lack of teeth, especially anterior teeth, malocclusion, drifting of teeth, diastemas between present teeth have negative impact on the oral health-related quality of life of the patients. Tooth agenesis poses medical problems due to ddysmorphic features that may only require cosmetic concern, or major anomalies that require clinical or cosmetic attention. Multidisciplinary teams[1] will manage therapeutic options, such as retaining the primary tooth, orthodontic treatment to close the edentulous spaces, dental surgical implants, and fixed or removable dental prosthetic appliances. The proper treatment may be tailored to the individual. It not only improves speech and masticatory function but also psychosocial distress that may help to restore self-confidence.

2. Terminology and classifications

There are several terms used to describe tooth agenesis: congenital absence of teeth, congenitally missing teeth, lack of teeth, or aplasia of teeth. Some suggest that the term" congenitally missing" teeth could be misleading because teeth are not visible at birth in the oral cavity and tooth development is completed after birth, or teeth may be lost by dental disease, or trauma, or extracted on clinical grounds. In the case of teeth, the development and differentiation continue long after birth, and instead of congenital many anomalies could rather be called developmental anomalies [3]. For the purpose of this chapter the term tooth agenesis will be used throughout. In the literature are used, most commonly, other descriptive terms mainly defined according to the number of missing teeth:

- Hypodontia is the lack of one to six teeth missing (excluding the third molars) with mild to moderate levels of severity.

---

[1] Clinical management of tooth agenesis requires careful multidisciplinary planning. Multidisciplinary team should include general dental practitioners, dental nurses, orthodontists, pedodontics, prosthodontists, oral and maxillofacial surgeons, specialist laboratory technicians, clinical psychologists, clinical geneticists, dermatologists, speech and language therapists.

- Oligodontia is the failure of development of more than six teeth missing (excluding the third molars) with severe level of severity.

- Anodontia means the lack of all teeth without any associated abnormalities causing an extremely severe dental phenotype.

The terms hypodontia and oligodontia are sometimes used interchangeably being considered as a unique clinical entity. As stated by Nieminen [3] and Vastardis [4], this classification of tooth agenesis may not properly reflect the severity of the phenotype as the third molars are excluded. Wherefore tooth agenesis based on dental phenotype severity may be partial or selective, or hypodontia (mild forms of agenesis), severe forms of agenesis or oligodontia, and very rare cases of agenesis of whole the dentition or anodontia. According to OMIM [5], selective tooth agenesis (STHAG) with no other associated systemic features or isolated tooth agenesis has been separated into two entities. The first entity refers to oligodontia characterized by the developmental absence of six or more permanent teeth. The second one refers to hypodontia characterized by the developmental failure of fewer than six teeth. The number of missing teeth in both cases excludes agenesis of third molars, commonly called wisdom teeth.

Incisor-premolar hypodontia (IPH) is a term also used in the literature based on the high frequency of incisors and premolars missing teeth [6]. For the purpose of this chapter the term tooth agenesis will be used throughout.

3. Clinical epidemiology

3.1 Prevalence of tooth agenesis

Prevalence of tooth agenesis is an important information to be of use not only for the clinician and patients but also for policy makers, given the implication for treatment protocols. Many published studies reported large variation in the prevalence of tooth agenesis across the world due to differences between methods of sampling, sample size, age of subjects, orthodontic or non-orthodontic enrolled subjects, number of males and females, the third molars included or excluded, or ethnic population groups. Moreover, it has been claimed that agenesis of permanent teeth has increased over the years. Mattheeuws et al. [7] considered that the period of time was too short and the available data too limited to describe a possible trend in the human dentition. Their meta-analysis seems to confirm that tooth agenesis has been diagnosed more often in recent studies.

Both the primary and permanent dentitions may be affected by variations in the number of teeth, but the prevalence is different. A prevalence of less than 1% in the primary dentition has been reported in the European population ranging from 0.4 to 0.9%, and it has been reported to be 2.4% in Japanese population [6, 8, 9].

Prevalence of permanent dentition has been studied extensively because it is no doubt more affected than primary dentition. Prevalence of tooth agenesis in permanent dentition also differs among studies of orthodontic/non-orthodontic subjects. Non-orthodontic population prevalence across the world varies between 1.6 and 9.6 per cent (most often-cited) [10–21] and calculated overall prevalence of tooth agenesis was estimated to be 6.53% $\pm$ 3.3% [22]. So far, some systematic reviews compare and evaluate prevalence studies on non-syndromic permanent teeth agenesis in various populations showing the prevalence varying from 0.3% in Indian population [16] to 15.7% in Hungarian population [17]. Polder et al. [11] reported the prevalence of non-syndromic agenesis in permanent teeth of European population (third molars excluded) varying between 3.4% in Switzerland to 10.1% in Norway. The wide range of prevalence values observed in population studies has suggested geographic differences. Published data reviewed by Pemberton et al. [23] reported that people of Scandinavian descent are the most susceptible to tooth agenesis in the permanent dentition whilst those of Asian or Arabic descent are the most susceptible in the primary dentition.

3.2 Distribution of tooth agenesis by gender

Gender predominance in tooth agenesis has been reported (**Table 1**) suggesting gender as a risk factor. Tooth agenesis show prevalence rates higher in females

Type of dentition	Prevalence %		Prevalence %	
	Minimum	Maximum	Male	Females
Primary	0.4	0.9	No significant differences	
Permanent	3.4	10.1	4.6	6.3

Table 1.
The prevalence of non-syndromic agenesis in permanent teeth (third molars excluded) in European population (summarized data).

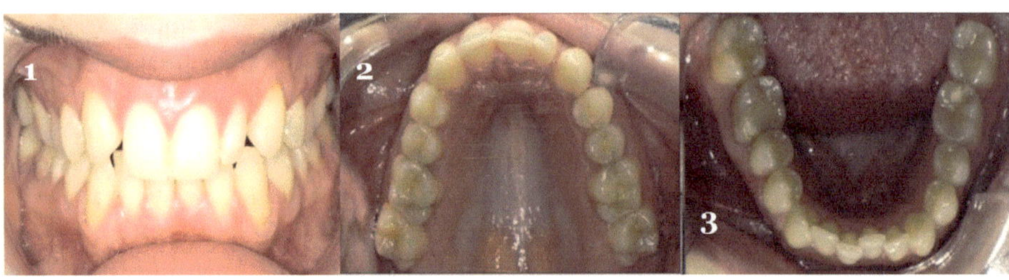

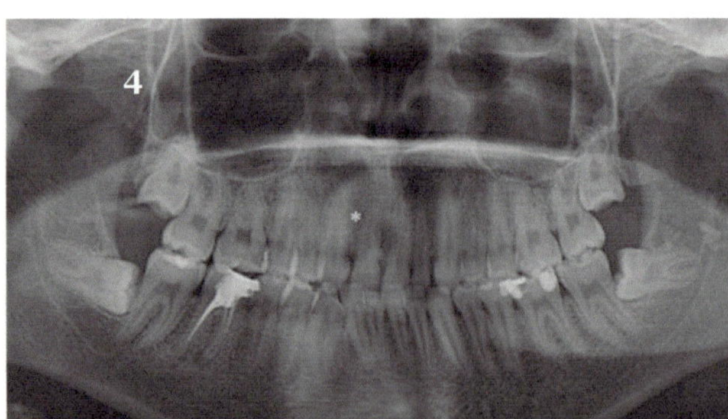

	Right quadrants	Left quadrants
Upper teeth (maxillary)	8 7 6 5 4 3 2* 1	1 2 3 4 5 6 7 8
Lower teeth (mandibular)	8 7 6 5 4 3 2 1	1 2 3 4 5 6 7 8

Figure 1.
*Female patient, 22 years old with non-syndromic tooth agenesis. (1,2,3) intraoral photos showing the missing upper right lateral incisor and the microdontia of the contralateral tooth. (4) panoramic radiograph confirming the agenesis of the maxillary right lateral incisor. * position of the missing tooth.*

compared to males [11, 12, 24]. However, other studies reported no significant difference between the prevalence of tooth agenesis in males and females [19, 20].

3.3 Number of missing teeth

In most patients, dental agenesis involved only one (47.8%) (**Figure 1**) or two teeth (35.1%) (**Figure 2**) [11]. Absence of one or two permanent teeth was reported in 83% - 87.9% of the subjects with tooth agenesis [11, 19, 20]. Thus, most of the affected individuals suffer only a mild form of tooth agenesis.

Although tooth agenesis is a common development anomaly, the prevalence becomes progressively smaller as the number of missing teeth increases. For example, isolated agenesis of at least six teeth is relatively rare, affecting 0.08% of the Dutch population [25] and 0.16% of the Danish population [26]. Polder et al. [11] reported an overall prevalence of 0.14% in affected patients with six or more teeth. In addition, lack of all teeth without associated abnormalities is extremely rare, and prevalence is unknown [19].

3.4 Tooth agenesis and type of teeth affected

Apparently, any tooth in the arch can be missing, but tooth agenesis tends to affect distinct tooth classes differentially. Some tooth types were more often

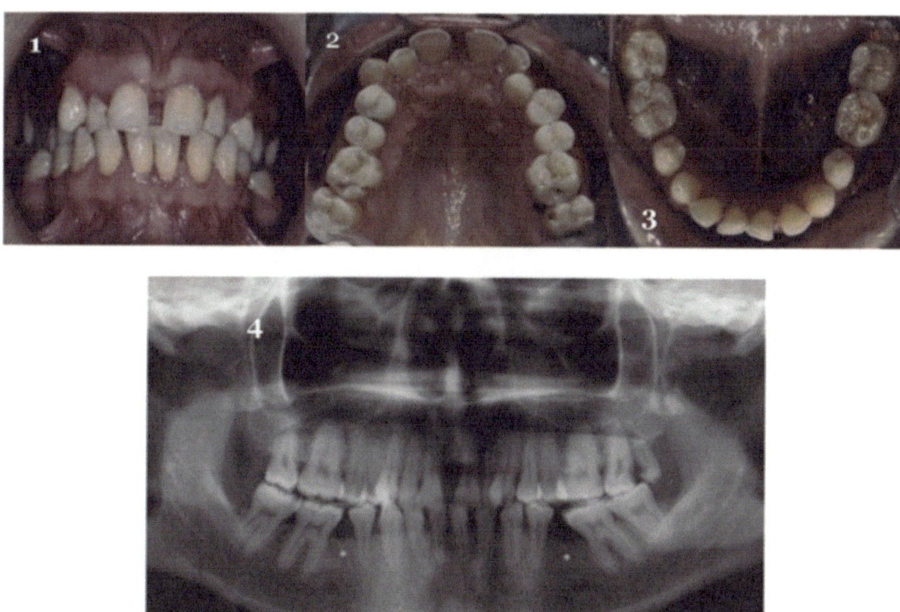

	Right quadrants	Left quadrants
Upper teeth (maxillary)	8 7 6 5 4 3 2 1	1 2 3 4 5 6 7 8
Lower teeth (mandibular)	8 7 6 5 4 3 2 1 *	1 2 3 4 5 6 7 8 *

Figure 2.
*A 28-year-old female patient with trisomy 21 presenting lower second premolars agenesis. Several dental anomalies are observed on the intraoral photos (1,2,3): Upper diastema, maxillary lateral incisors microdontia, ectopic canines and spaced lower teeth. (4) panoramic radiograph shows the absence of the lower second premolars and an agenesis diagnosis can be confirmed. * position of the missing tooth.*

missing than other ones. Thus, the frequency of the individual teeth involved varies [11].

In the deciduous dentition, the upper lateral incisors account for more than 50% and together with lower incisors for 90% of all affected teeth [27]. Nieminen highlighted that there is an obvious association between the agenesis of the temporary teeth and the permanent teeth; a temporary tooth affected by agenesis is almost every time followed by missing of the corresponding permanent tooth [3, 27].

The third molars are the most prevalent missing teeth in all reports. Up to 70% of the population experience problems with their third molars, whether it is failure of proper eruption (impaction) or not erupting at all (agenesis). Up to 25% of the population may lose at least one third molar [10] and therefore, usually, third molar is excluded from the classification. The lowest prevalence of third molar agenesis reported so far was 10.1% for African American population [28] and the highest prevalence was 41% for the Korean population [29]. Excluding the third molars, in European population, the most frequently missing tooth is mandibular second premolar (2.91%–3.22%), followed by maxillary lateral incisor (1.55%–1.78%) or second premolar (1.39%–1.61%), as reviewed by Gracco et al. [19].

Other data support the conclusion that the most commonly missing tooth was the maxillary lateral incisor, followed by mandibular and maxillary second premolars [22]. **Figure 3** illustrates the bilateral absence of second lower premolars. Agenesis of lower central incisors is common in Asian populations in both primary and permanent dentitions [9].

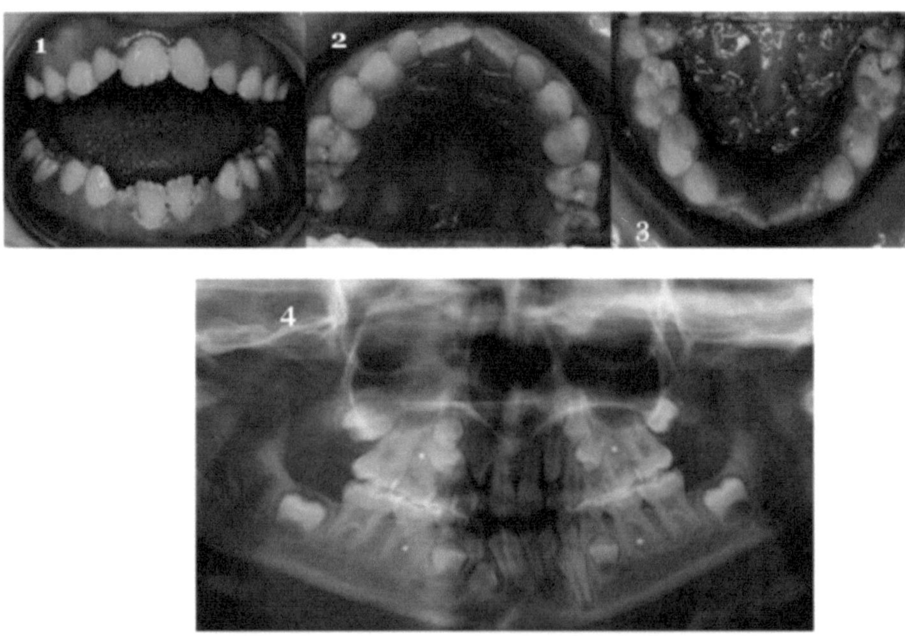

	Right quadrants	Left quadrants
Upper teeth (maxillary)	* 8 7 6 5 4 3 2 1	* 1 2 3 4 5 6 7 8
Lower teeth (mandibular)	8 7 6 5 4 3 2 1 *	1 2 3 4 5 6 7 8 *

Figure 3.
Female patient aged 7 years old with confirmed trisomy 21 presenting all four second premolars agenesis. Intraoral photos (1,2,3) emphasize a mixed dentition with lack of space for the alignment of the permanent teeth. (4) panoramic radiograph shows the congenital absence of the second premolars in both dental arches.
** position of the missing tooth.*

Less commonly affected teeth are, in order, lower incisors, maxillary first premolars, mandibular first premolars, maxillary canines and mandibular second molars (**Figure 4**). Patients who experience agenesis of these teeth (e.g., canine or maxillary central incisor) more often present with many missing teeth [11].

The most stable teeth are maxillary central incisors (prevalence of agenesis 0.016%) and mandibular first molars and canines (prevalence of agenesis about 0.03%) [3]. Recently, Eshgian et al. [21] concluded that hypodontia affected specific type of teeth. In their study, the most commonly missing teeth were maxillary premolars, lateral incisors and mandibular premolars. Comparing their results with other data from previous studies, they explained the differences in patterns and prevalence of tooth agenesis between different population groups by ethnic diversity in the distributions of mutant genes. The explanation was supported by the prevalence of people with missing permanent teeth which was significantly lower in blacks than in whites in U.S.A. [28], and different type of affected tooth, mandibular incisor in Hong Kong children population [30] and mandibular second premolars among Italians [19]. Polder et al. [11] considered that difference in the ethnic groups is not the explanation of differences in prevalence between populations due to the small number of reported hypodontia cases and the difficulty of detecting the anomaly without appropriate evidence.

Distinct patterns of permanent teeth agenesis have been reported but, as a general rule, if only one or a few teeth are missing, the absent tooth will be the most distal tooth of any given morphological class [3, 15, 24, 31].

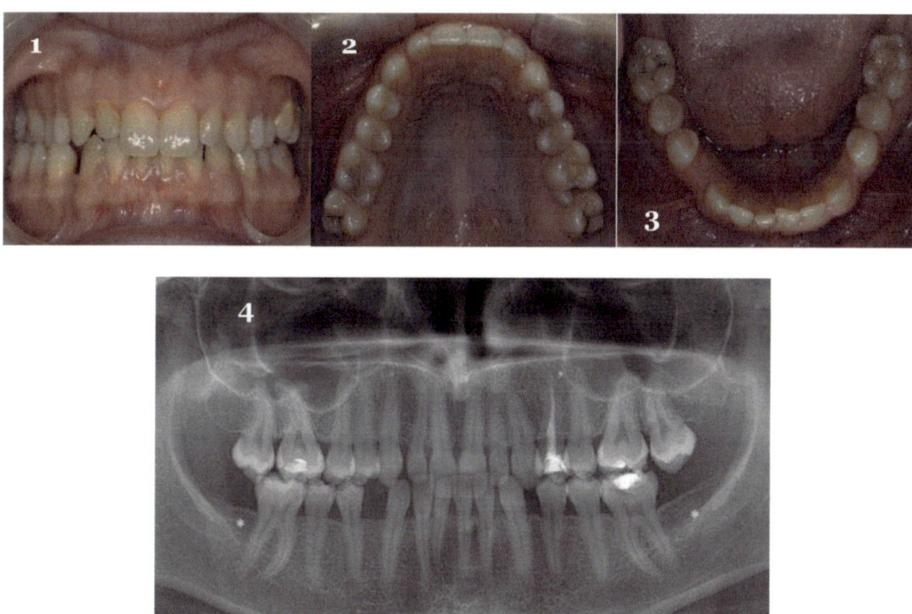

	Right quadrants	Left quadrants
Upper teeth (maxillary)	8 7 6 5 4 3 2 1	1 2 3 4 5 6 7 8
Lower teeth (mandibular)	8 7 6 5 4 3 2 1 * (under 7)	1 2 3 4 5 6 7 8 * (under 7)

Figure 4.
*Tooth agenesis in a non-syndromic 21-year-old female patient. Intraoral photos (1,2,3) emphasizing a generalized microdontia and as a result, teeth are spaced with larger gaps in the lower arch. (4) Anamnesis and the examination of the panoramic x-ray reveal the congenital absence of the lower second molars, both in the right and in the left quadrant. * position of the missing teeth.*

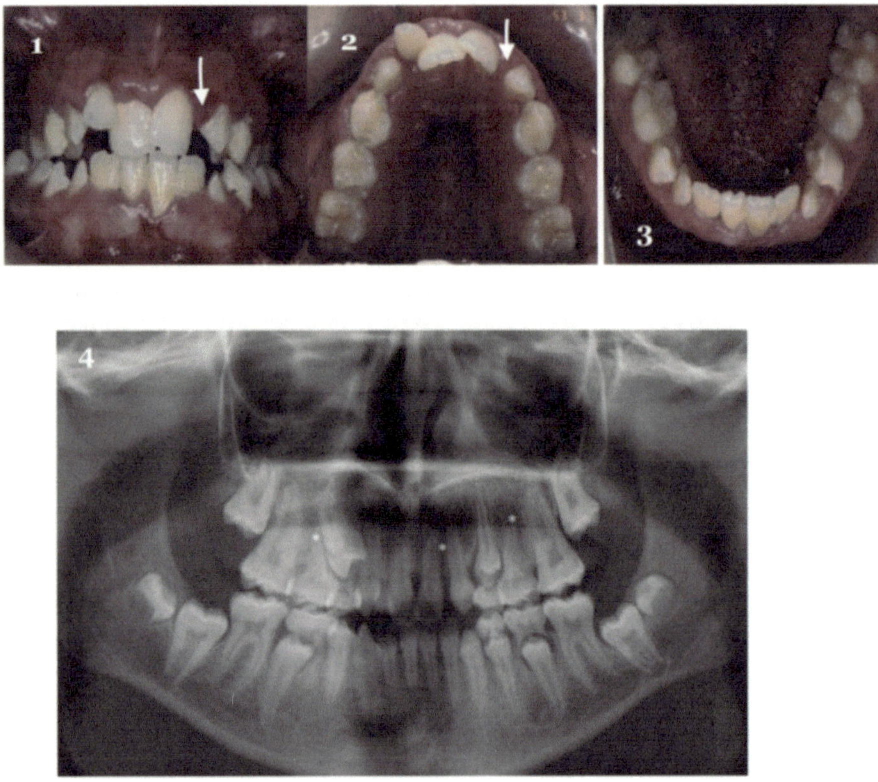

	Right quadrants	Left quadrants
Upper teeth (maxillary)	* 8 7 6 5 4 3 2 1	* * 1 2 3 4 5 6 7 8
Lower teeth (mandibular)	8 7 6 5 4 3 2 1	1 2 3 4 5 6 7 8

Figure 5.
*A 13-year-old male with confirmed Down syndrome presenting different dental anomalies. Intraoral photos (1–3) show mixed dentition with delayed eruption of permanent teeth, remarking the absence of the upper left lateral incisor. (4) Examination of the panoramic radiograph reveals the absence of the upper second premolars and of the maxillary left lateral incisor. * position of the missing teeth.*

It is known that upper lateral incisors, second premolars, and third molars are the last forming teeth in their tooth family, are in the embryonic fusion of the maxilla and the medial nasal processes and erupt in the critical terminal area of the dental lamina. For these reasons, the last forming teeth are more vulnerable to the critical actions of both genetic and environmental factors during odontogenesis and fail to develop. This can explain why tooth agenesis most frequently affects premolars, lateral incisors, and molars (**Figure 5**). The anomaly was called ‘end-of-series [31, 32]. In 2017, it has been assumed by Juuri and Balic that tooth agenesis most frequently affects the last tooth to develop within the tooth family due to a gradual decrease of the odontogenic potential of the dental lamina [33].

3.5 Bilateral versus unilateral tooth agenesis

Tooth agenesis may be either bilateral or unilateral. Pinho et al. [32] hypothesized that if the etiology of hypodontia is primarily genetic, then bilateral missing teeth phenotype would be expected to be more commonly observed. Unilateral hypodontia might be a variation in severity of a genetic trait showing a microdont or peg-shaped contralateral tooth.

Most studies reported predominance of bilateral missing teeth, as reviewed by Rakhshan [15]. Goya et al. [34] found that symmetry of congenitally missing teeth was predominant (74.6%), Kirzioglu et al. [35] observed that bilaterally missing teeth was 73.2%, and Endo et al. [36] reported that 89% of the patients presented bilaterally missing teeth. Other researchers have found unilateral tooth agenesis more common [37]. Polder et al. [11] compared (based on nine studies) the occurrence of bilateral and unilateral agenesis for the most four affected teeth showing that only for maxillary lateral incisors prevalence of unilateral agenesis was lower than bilateral agenesis.

- Bilateral agenesis of maxillary lateral incisors occurred more often.
- Unilateral agenesis involving mandibular second premolars occurred more common.
- Unilateral agenesis affecting maxillary second premolars was more frequently.
- Unilateral agenesis of mandibular central incisors occurred more often.

Medina [38] stated that while symmetrical dental missing affects the maxilla (**Figure 6**), the mandible shows mostly unilateral agenesis. In the opinion of other

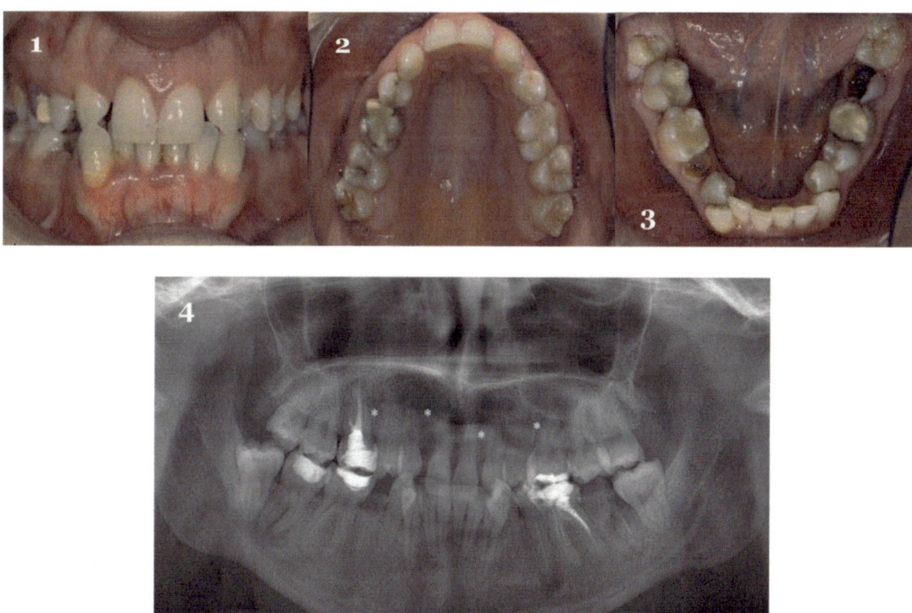

	Right quadrants	Left quadrants
Upper teeth (maxillary)	* * 8 7 6 5 4 3 2 1	* * 1 2 3 4 5 6 7 8
Lower teeth (mandibular)	8 7 6 5 4 3 2 1	1 2 3 4 5 6 7 8

Figure 6.
*Non-syndromic tooth agenesis in a 26-year-old female patient. Clinical intraoral appearance (1,2,3) emphasizing multiple dental problems, accentuated by the bilateral absence of the upper lateral incisors and of the second premolars. (4) panoramic radiograph confirming the agenesis of the four upper teeth. * position of the missing teeth.*

researchers, the most common symmetric missing tooth could be the mandibular second premolar agenesis, followed by the absence of the maxillary second premolar or maxillary lateral incisor, as reviewed by Rakhshan [15].

3.6 Distribution of missing teeth over maxilla/mandible

No overall difference in tooth agenesis has been reported between maxilla and mandible for permanent dentition [11]. However, Gomes et al. [20] found maxillary hypodontia in 59.2% of patients and in the mandible of 40.8% with an overall ratio of 1.45:1 in orthodontic patients. Several reports mentioned a small but not always significant predominance of missing teeth in the maxilla [19, 20, 24] whilst other reported more missing teeth in the mandible than in the maxilla [36].

For the primary teeth, agenesis is more common in the maxilla [27].

3.7 Distribution of missing teeth over left/right sides

No significant difference between left and right sides of the jaw has been reported. Nevertheless, predominance of tooth agenesis on the left side has been reported in some Scandinavian studies, as reviewed by Arte S. [18] and Fekonja A. [24] have found the missing teeth were more commonly absent on the right side.

3.8 Distribution of missing teeth across anterior/posterior regions

No clear difference in tooth agenesis has been found between the anterior and posterior regions. Most studies showed higher prevalence in the anterior segment [15] and the few remaining analyses found no significant differences [36]. Endo et al. [36] suggested that in mild cases of tooth agenesis, the anterior segment might be more involved while the posterior segment might be predominant in severe cases.

3.9 Age of detectability

Polder et al. considered the age of detectability as an important issue. A meta-analysis study made by Polder et al. revealed that the visibility of tooth germs by X-ray examination hangs on their degree of mineralization. Subjects at the same chronological age can show significant differences in mineralization stages and dental age. The major differences in mineralization can be found especially in mandibular second premolar buds or third molar buds which present a late onset of mineralization. Therefore, radiographic examination may show a false-positive result and a misdiagnosis of tooth agenesis [11].

All primary teeth have erupted by the age of three and all permanent teeth except the third molars between the age of 12 and 14. Therefore, three to four years of age children are suitable for diagnosis of missing primary teeth by clinical examination, and 12 to 14-year-old children (the precise determination of teeth mineralization stages), for diagnosis of permanent teeth [22, 39]. While some studies reported age of detectability after eight years of age for the permanent dentition, and failure for the third molar to form is detectable by age 11.

4. Genetic causes of tooth agenesis

Investigations so far show that several heterogenous factors may be involved in tooth agenesis. Tooth development is a complex process which involves a combination of genetic, epigenetic, and environmental factors. Thus, there is no single etiology of tooth agenesis. Family, twin, and adoption studies[2] are the primary exploration by which the genetic basis of a condition may be established. In addition, observed prevalence differences between populations, and association with heritable syndromes supplied evidence for strong genetic influences on tooth agenesis [8]. These findings provided the reasoning for recent efforts to identify the relevant susceptibility genes and the molecular mechanisms by which they interact with environmental influences, and to correlate tooth agenesis phenotypes with their causative factors. Furthermore, genetic studies on mouse models with dental agenesis have identified a few transcription factors and signaling molecules, such as WNTs (wingless-related integration site), BMPs (bone morphogenetic proteins), FGFs (fibroblast growth factor), and NF–κB (nuclear factor kappa B) as candidate genes in human isolated and syndromic agenesis [40].

More than 300 genes are expressed and control odontogenesis and, apparently, any of these gene mutations may cause tooth agenesis. Among these genes, PAX9 (paired box gene 9), MSX1 (muscle segment homeobox 1), EDA (ectodysplasin A), WNT10A (wingless-type MMTV integration site family, member 10A), and AXIN2 (axis inhibitor 2) are the most frequently reported mutations associated with non-syndromic tooth agenesis (hypodontia/oligodontia), as reviewed by Al-Ani et al. [41] and Liu et al. [42]. (**Table 2**) These all genes have roles in both signaling pathways and in mediating the signal transduction cascades.

Normal expression of these genes is important for the tooth development. MSX1 is a transcription factors active in regions of condensing ectomesenchyme in the tooth germ. PAX9 is a transcription factor as well, it is expressed in the tooth mesenchyme, playing a significant role during odontogenesis in the progressive and reciprocal signal transduction pathways that normally occur in epithelial–mesenchymal cells. Both Msx1 and Pax9 are involved in the Bmp and Fgf pathways and interact during the tooth-bud-to-cap transition. Their expression profiles during early tooth development are largely overlapping, and Pax9 is known to activate transcription of *Msx1* at the bud stage. AXIN2 plays an important role in the regulation of the stability of beta-catenin in the Wnt signaling pathway. EDA is involved in epithelial-mesenchymal signaling during morphogenesis of ectodermal organs, including teeth, hairs, feathers, and mammary glands. WNT10A is strongly expressed in the dental epithelium at the initiation stage and plays a role in tooth development beyond the bud stage [31].

Studying 34 unrelated patients with isolated tooth agenesis, van den Boogaard et al. [43] reported that 19 patients, representing 56% of them, had mutations in the WNT10A gene. Of 34 patients, 3% presented mutations in the MSX1 gene, 9% and 3% had mutations in the PAX9 and AXIN2 genes, respectively. It was concluded that WNT10A is a significant gene in the etiology of isolated hypodontia.

Frameshift and nonsense mutations are highly likely all causative because they involve profound alteration of the protein primary structure, but missense mutations in these genes are found to cause tooth agenesis phenotypes characteristic in terms of severity and affected teeth as well [44].

---

[2] If a tooth agenesis is caused by genetic factors, then individuals who are genetically related should share similar risks for the condition. Family studies look for genes that cause familial aggregation of a heritable trait. Twin studies compare the rate of tooth agenesis between monozygotic and dizygotic twins as a test for genetic contributions. Monozygotic twins have been concordant and have shown variation due to epigenetic factors, environmental modifiers, or interactions. Studies of adoption can help distinguish the relative influence of genes and environment.

Gene symbol/ locus	Gene name	Cytogenetic location	Gene / locus OMIM number	Description of tooth agenesis clinical features	Inheritance	Phenotype OMIM Number
AXIN2	axis inhibitor 2	17q24.1	604025	Oligodontia – severe permanent teeth agenesis	Autosomal DOMINANT	608615
EDA	ectodysplasin A	Xq13.1	300451	Tooth agenesis, selective, X-linked 1 (STHAGX1)	X-linked DOMINANT	313500
GREM2	GREMLIN-2 homolog, cystine knot superfamily gene	1q43	608832	Tooth agenesis, selective,9 (STHAG9)	Autosomal DOMINANT	617275
LRP6	low density lipoprotein receptor-related protein-6	12p13.2	603507	Tooth agenesis, selective,7 (STHAG7)	Autosomal DOMINANT	616724
MSX1	muscle segment homeobox 1	4p16.2	142983	Tooth agenesis, selective,1, with or without orofacial cleft (STHAG1)	Autosomal DOMINANT	106600
PAX9	paired box gene 9	14q13.3	167416	Tooth agenesis, selective,3 (STHAG3) Hypodontia/ Oligodontia 3	Autosomal DOMINANT	604625
STHAG2		16q12.1* (*the disorder was placed on the map by statistical methods)	602639	Tooth agenesis, selective, (STHAG2)	Autosomal recessive	602639
STHAG5		10q11.2-q21* (*the disorder was placed on the map by statistical methods)	610926	Tooth agenesis, selective,5 (STHAG5) Hypodontia/ Oligodontia 5 (He-Zhao deficiency)		610926
WNT10A	wingless-type MMTV integration site family, member 10A	2q35	606268	Tooth agenesis, selective,4 (STHAG4) with or without ectodermal dysplasia	Autosomal DOMINANT or recessive	150400
WNT10B	wingless-type MMTV integration site family, member-10B	12q13.12	601906	Tooth agenesis, selective,8 (STHAG8)	Autosomal DOMINANT	617073

Online Mendelian Inheritance in Man (OMIM™) is a comprehensive, authoritative and timely knowledgebase of human genes and genetic phenotype compiled to support research and education in human genomics and the practice of clinical genetics. It is freely available and updated daily.

Table 2.
Gene mutations involved in NON-SYNDROMIC tooth agenesis are passed on to the next generation following different Mendelian patterns of inheritance (according to OMIM database).

As a rule, homozygous (identical mutation on both alleles of a specific gene) or compound heterozygous (both alleles of a gene are mutant, but the mutations are different) carriers of gene mutations exhibit more severe phenotype of tooth agenesis than heterozygous carriers (two different alleles, but only one is mutant).

Besides the single-gene mutations, Michon [45] reported the functional role of miRNAs in proliferation and differentiation of cells and tissues during odontogenesis and possible dental defects development. His results support the view of complex genetic etiology of tooth agenesis.

Attention should be turned to the expression of a mutation in a family. In families with a probable dominant or recessive Mendelian inheritance, there seems to be a variable missing teeth phenotype. In other words, tooth agenesis patterns are different in expressivity among the affected members within a family having the same molecular cause. Vastardis studied incisor agenesis in families with dominant pattern of inheritance. Autosomal dominant disorders express variability in clinical manifestation caused by reduced penetrance and variable expressivity of mutant gene. Consequently, individuals in the same family who carry an identical mutation can vary in the severity of their incisor agenesis. Variable expressivity determines developmental alteration of lateral incisor shape (peg-shaped) or rudimentary third molars and unilateral agenesis may be the result of incomplete penetrance [46].

Mostowska et al. described a three-generation family with severe autosomal dominant oligodontia. Those affected lacked all permanent molars, second premolars, and mandibular central incisors. The authors found a novel mutation of MSX1. Mutation occurs in exon 2, at nucleotide 581 a cytosine is changed to a thymine (c.581C $\rightarrow$ T transition), and disrupts the homeobox domain, which is highly conserved. The new mutation causes non-syndromic oligodontia (absence of 14 permanent teeth) in their proband. Two healthy members from the proband's family carry the same missense mutation [47]. To date, many studies provide evidence for great intra- and inter-familial clinical variability in families with isolated tooth agenesis [3, 13, 41].

There are several possible genetic mechanisms to explain these major differences in expressivity of the phenotype with the same molecular cause. One of them lies in the concepts of penetrance and expressivity. Reduced (incomplete) penetrance and variable expressivity are factors that influence the effects of particular genetic changes and are commonly seen with Mendelian dominant traits. Tooth agenesis shows incomplete penetrance, since pedigree studies demonstrate individuals who must carry the mutation but who do not appear to be affected themselves. Reduced penetrance probably occurs when final effect of a gene mutation can be indirectly influenced by modifier genes, epigenetic factors, or miRNAs. Potential modifier genes may act in the same or in different development pathways altering (exacerbate or attenuate the effect of the gene mutation) the clinical phenotype.

Epigenetic factors do not change the gene sequence. Epigenetic alterations may be induced spontaneously, in response to environmental factors, or may be part of a person's make up (allele dosage, copy number variants, allele variants). Identical twins are ideal subjects for studying the effects of epigenetic modifications. Monozygotic co-twins sharing sex, age, and identical genomes display discordant phenotypes for missing teeth which may be explained by epigenetic differences. In their twin study, Townsend et al. supported the view that, even though there is a relatively strong genetic basis to missing teeth, the number or position of affected teeth can be influenced by epigenetic factors. Epigenetic alteration activities, such as DNA methylation and histone modification, at each stage, at the local level during the odontogenesis process, may account for distinct phenotypic differences in the final appearance of teeth of the identical twins. During tooth development, odontogenetic cells reply differently to epigenetic variation in spatiotemporal expression of local signaling molecules passing between cells. [48]

miRNAs play an important role in controlling gene activity by regulating translation during tooth development. Changes in miRNAs levels have been linked to several dental defects [45]. Thus, in a population, the missing teeth phenotype might not occur so often as the abnormal genotype. On the other hand, individuals with the same genetic condition may have more missing teeth than another having only one missing tooth. Thus, expressivity describes individual variability. Variable expressivity is probably caused by a combination of genetic, environmental, and lifestyle factors, most of which have not been identified.

Dreesen et al. analyzed hypo−/oligodontia phenotype variations in nine families at individual, intrafamilial and interfamilial levels aiming to evaluate whether the different agenesis patterns in the pedigrees are predictive of mutations in specific genes based on reported genotype–phenotype associations. Familial aggregation was noted but the tooth agenesis patterns were variable between family members, in terms of number of missing teeth. Therefore, tooth agenesis is not (always) a simple monogenic disorder. The authors proposed a multifactorial aetiological model with many genes and environmental factors modulating the clinical expression [49].

4.1 Genetic heterogeneity of selective tooth agenesis (STHAG) and clinical features

Genetic heterogeneity describes different gene mutations or genetic mechanisms that produce the same or similar clinical phenotype. Heterogeneity can be recognized by subtle differences in clinical phenotype or evidence of different patterns of inheritance. Genetic testing can confirm the gene mutation responsible for a certain clinical phenotype. Usually, genetic heterogeneity complicates the risk estimation in genetic counseling and genetic prognoses.

Two types of genetic heterogeneity are recognized: locus heterogeneity (clinical phenotype is caused by mutations at two or more different loci), and allelic heterogeneity (clinical phenotype is caused by more than one mutation within the same gene, same locus).

Locus heterogeneity is well documented in selective tooth agenesis (STHAG).

There are ten loci associated with STHAG. Nine of them are autosomal loci (STHAG1 to STHAG9) and one STHAGX1 is sex-linked locus as it follows the X-linked dominant pattern of inheritance. The corresponding gene located at **STAHG1** is MSX1 on chromosome 4p16. The genes for the following loci are PAX9-**STHAG3** on chromosome 14q12, WNT10A-**STHAG4** on chromosome 2q35, formerly LTB3-**STHAG6** on chromosome 11q13.1, LRP6-**STHAG7** on chromosome 12p13, WNT10B-**STHAG8** on chromosome 12q13, GREM2-**STHAG9** on chromosome 1q43, and EDA-**STHAGX1** on chromosome Xq13. The molecular basis of STHAG is known for STHAG1,3,4,7,9 and STHAHX1. For STHAG2 and 5, the disorder was placed on the map by statistical methods. (**Table 2**).

In 1998, Ahmad et al. [50] reported an autosomal recessive form of hypodontia in a large consanguineous Pakistani family. This was the first report of hypodontia associated with other dental anomalies, such as enamel hypoplasia and failure of teeth eruption, leading to the edentulous state prematurely. The locus was named **STHAG2** which is located on chromosome 16p12, but the gene for this locus has not been described so far.

In 2000, Wang et al. [51] described a rare, heritable, form of agenesis of permanent teeth. The tooth number anomaly was named He-Zhao deficiency. The only clinical feature of affected individuals was oligodontia. It was transmitted in an autosomal dominant manner with reduced penetrance in a large six successive generation family coming from a small village in China. The number of missing teeth ranged from "a few teeth to the entire set of teeth". Some of the patients were more likely to have first and second molars. This distinct form of permanent tooth agenesis is associated with **STHAG5** locus on chromosome 10q11.2.

In 2015, Huckert et al. [52] reported mutations in LTBP3 (latent transforming growth factor-beta-binding protein 3) gene causing different dental phenotypes and brachyolmia (short trunk, mild short stature with platyspondyly and scoliosis). The association of oligodontia with hypoplastic amelogenesis imperfecta, taurodontic molars and short stature has been designed as a distinct entity named DASS (dental anomalies and short stature) (OMIM 601216). So, STHAG6 was incorporated into DASS.

Another example of locus heterogeneity is provided by mutations in EDA, EDAR and EDARADD genes which express the similar phenotype of hypohidrotic ectodermal dysplasia (**Table 3**).

Allelic heterogeneity is illustrated by the different mutations in the MSX1 and PAX9 genes. For example, MSX1 mutations show overlapping and non-overlapping phenotypes. Almost all mutations are responsible for autosomal dominant STHAG1 involving second premolars, first molars and third molars. Few MSX1 mutations are associated with combinations of tooth agenesis with oral clefting (cleft palate only and cleft lip and cleft palate) and nail abnormalities (Witkop syndrome) [49] (**Table 3**).

4.2 Genotype–phenotype correlations

Genotype–phenotype correlations refer to the association between specific germline mutations, meaning genotype, and the resulting spectrum of disease expression of that mutation in the affected individual, meaning phenotype. Usually, such correlations are made for monogenic disorders which follow Mendelian inheritance patterns. Moreover, the correlations can clarify which characteristics of a mutation affect the severity of dental anomaly with a genetic background. On the other hand, the pattern of tooth agenesis provides useful information about how gene mutation might affect an individual and other member of the family. Tooth agenesis runs in families and hypodontia/oligodontia patients have one or more affected family members [48]. So, the family members can be appropriately counseled by a geneticist, and predictive/pre-symptomatic genetic testing should be considered for early diagnosis and early intervention, especially for children.

Research studies have linked non-syndromic hypodontia/oligodontia phenotype with specific gene mutations. For example, among identified mutations, MSX1 and PAX9 genes can cause variation in clinical phenotype of tooth agenesis. Kim et al. [53] studied the pattern of missing teeth in families with certain MSX1 and PAX9 mutations. The missing teeth pattern associated with MSX1 mutants was different from that associated with mutations in PAX9. MSX1-associated tooth agenesis involved bilaterally symmetrical absence of maxillary and mandibular second premolars and maxillary first premolars. PAX9-associated tooth agenesis involved also bilaterally symmetrical missing teeth, usually maxillary and mandibular second molars were affected. Yu et al. [54] stated that WNTB10B-associated oligodontia affected most lateral incisors. In contrast, genotype–phenotype analysis of oligodontia pattern associated with WNT10A mutations revealed that premolars were the most frequently missing teeth.

4.3 Familial non-syndromic severe tooth agenesis (oligodontia)

Mutations in nine genes (MSX1, PAX9, AXIN2, WNT10A, EDA, EDAR, EDARADD, NEMO and KRT17) have been associated with non-syndromic

Gene symbol	Gene name	Cytogenetic location	Gene/locus OMIM number	Name of disorder associated with tooth agenesis	Inheritance	Phenotype OMIM Number
AXIN2	axis inhibitor 2	17q24.1	604025	Oligodontia-colorectal cancer syndrome	Autosomal DOMINANT	608615
EDA	ectodysplasin A	Xq13.1	300451	Hypohidrotic ectodermal dysplasia 1 (HED)	X-linked reccessive	305100
EDAR	ectodysplasin A receptor	2q13	604095	Ectodermal dysplasia 10A, hypohidrotic/hair/nail type Ectodermal dysplasia 10B, hypohidrotic/hair/nail type	Autosomal DOMINANT Autosomal recessive	129490 224900
EDARADD	edar-associated death domain	1q42-q43	606603	Ectodermal dysplasia 11A, hypohidrotic/hair/tooth type Ectodermal dysplasia 11B, hypohidrotic/hair/tooth type	Autosomal DOMINANT Autosomal recessive	614940 614941
LTBP3	latent transforming growth factor-beta-binding protein 3	11q13.1	602090	Dental anomalies and short stature	Autosomal recessive	601216
MSX1	muscle segment homeobox 1	4p16.2	142983	Ectodermal dysplasia 3, Witkop type Orofacial cleft 5 Wolf-Hirschhorn syndrome* (*a contiguous gene deletion syndrome in which multiple genes are involved)	Autosomal DOMINANT Autosomal DOMINANT Isolated cases	189500 608874 194190
NEMO (IKBKG)	inhibitor of nuclear factor kappa-b kinase, regulatory subunit gamma	xq28	300248	Incontinentia pigmenti	X-linked DOMINANT	308300
PITX2	paired-like homeodomain transcription factor 2	4q25	601542	Axenfeld-Rieger syndrome, type 1	Autosomal DOMINANT	180500
WNT10A	wingless-type MMTV integration site family, member 10A	2q35	606268	Schopf-Schulz-Passarge syndrome Odontoonychodermal dysplasia	Autosomal recessive Autosomal recessive	224750 257980

Table 3.
Gene mutations frequently associated with SYNDROMIC tooth agenesis.

oligodontia, as reviewed by Liu et al. [42] Oligodontia phenotype is caused by haploinsufficiency. Mutations produce a reduction in functional gene product below a threshold required for normal dental development [8].

Apparently, reduced quantities of a gene product should equally affect the formation of all teeth. Oligodontia caused by defects in MSX1 and PAX9 yields typical, although variable and overlapping patterns of tooth agenesis [8]. Mutations of MSX1 result in the absence of all permanent third molars, all second premolars, maxillary first premolars and variably other teeth, whereas defects in PAX9 cause mainly agenesis of molars, typically of all permanent maxillary and the second and third mandibular molars as well as variably of other teeth [55]. Regarding AXIN2 gene, five mutations were reported to be associated with non-syndromic tooth agenesis: four missense and one frameshift mutations. The phenotype is variable in expression and involved at least seven teeth. One study reported that a mutation in EDARADD gene led to non-syndromic oligodontia [41].

4.4 Tooth agenesis as a complex (multifactorial) trait

Not all of the tooth agenesis forms can be linked to precis genetic mutations, at a single gene locus. Tooth agenesis is a common developmental anomaly and has a definite familial tendency. However, the proportion of affected near relatives is less than what expected for a monogenic trait. One way to recognize a complex trait is through unpredictable inheritance patterns in successive generations. Tooth agenesis is probably caused by several independent defective genes, acting alone or in combination with other genes, and interacting with environmental factors, leading to a specific clinical phenotypic pattern. Being produced by multiple genes, a multifactorial trait seems to be more susceptible to environmental/stochastic or nongenetic factors.

Incomplete penetrance, genetic background, and variable expression levels did not explain all major differences in the expressivity of the phenotype with the same molecular cause. For these reasons, some authors based on evidence from genetic studies, animal models, and environmental correlates suggested an oligogenic or polygenic inheritance of tooth agenesis [42, 45–48].

For instance, Vastardis [45] stated that tooth development is a very complex process and involves many" players". Thus, third molar agenesis cannot be explained in most cases with a simple model of autosomal dominant transmission. Fekonja et al. [24] suggested that genes could be the dominant factor for the agenesis in the anterior region, while the posterior teeth could be missing sporadically. Townsend et al. [56] proposed a multifactorial aetiological model, with possibly many genes, and also environmental and epigenetic factors contributing to tooth development based on lack of complete concordance for missing teeth in monozygotic twins.

It has been documented by various statistical analyses using single locus and polygenic patterns that both approaches are possible. From genetical point of view, multifactorial inheritance of tooth agenesis is troublesome to analyze. It is difficult to state whether hypodontia is a result of a polygenic or single gene defect. It arrives at a diagnosis of multifactorial inheritance for tooth agenesis only after the monogenic forms of inheritance have been considered and found unlikely.

4.5 Familial non-syndromic permanent teeth anodontia

Molecular basis or locus of isolated anodontia (OMIM 206780) are unknown. Gorlin et al. [57] described complete absence of the permanent dentition with the entire primary dentition present and erupted at a normal time. Anodontia presented evidence of autosomal recessive inheritance, including multiple affected sibs and consanguineous parents. Based on three family studies, it was documented that anodontia of permanent teeth is a homozygous state of the gene responsible for pegged or missing maxillary lateral incisors [5].

Pseudoanodontia should not be confused with anodontia. Pseudoanodontia or false anodontia occurs, when teeth are absent clinically because of impaction, delayed eruption, exfoliation or extraction. In GAPO syndrome (GAPO syndrome is the acronymic designation for a complex of growth retardation, alopecia, pseudoanodontia, and progressive optic atrophy - OMIM 230740) is described pseudoanodontia, failure of tooth eruption. The syndrome is caused by mutations of ANTXR1 gene (anthrax toxin receptor 1) located on 2p13.3, and the pattern of inheritance is autosomal recessive [58].

4.6 Syndromic tooth agenesis

Tooth agenesis is usually isolated, but gene mutations have been identified that either cause tooth agenesis as a sole isolated agenesis, or tooth agenesis in association with a wide variety of multiorgan malformation syndromes. (**Table 3 and Appendix 1 – Table A1**)) The London dysmorphology database reported 150 syndromes as being associated with hypodontia [18].

Thus, tooth agenesis is a primary feature of many single-gene Mendelian syndromes that affect not only teeth but also several other ectodermal derivatives indicating that the development of teeth and certain tissues/organs are under the control of the same gene molecular functions and common molecular mechanisms are responsible for tooth and other organ development. A pleiotropic mutation may influence several, apparently unrelated, traits simultaneously, due to the gene coding for a product used by a myriad of cells or different targets that have the same signaling function. For instance, two AXIN2 nonsense mutations caused syndromic tooth agenesis, such as oligodontia and predispose to colorectal cancer, or oligodontia and variable other findings, including colonic polyposis, gastric polyps, a mild ectodermal dysplasia phenotype with sparse hair and eyebrows, and early onset colorectal and breast cancers [42].

Adventitious chromosomal abnormalities cause tooth agenesis in association with other clinical features and recognizable patterns of malformations known as chromosomal syndromes.

- Down syndrome and tooth agenesis (OMIM 190685)

  Down syndrome (DS), a common and well-known syndrome, is caused by an autosomal aneuploid defect called trisomy involving the human chromosome 21 (Ts21). The extra chromosome 21 or part of its long arm (including many genes) may come in distinct genetic ways, such as full trisomy 21, mosaic trisomy 21 or unbalanced translocation trisomy 21 causing DS distinctive facial features. The difference between DS people could be made by chromosome analysis because craniofacial features are similar. So, cytogenetic analysis is not relevant for predicting the severity of oro-dental features in DS [59].

  Missing teeth were reported in 23–47% of cases (**Figure 7**). Third molars, second premolars, and lateral incisors are most frequently absent in the permanent dentition. Peg-shaped maxillary lateral incisors have been observed in 10%. In 12–17% of cases, deciduous lateral incisors are missing. Extreme hypodontia and anodontia have been noted occasionally [60]. There is a higher incidence of dental anomalies, such as taurodontism, fusion of deciduous lower lateral incisor with a canine, morphologic crown alterations,

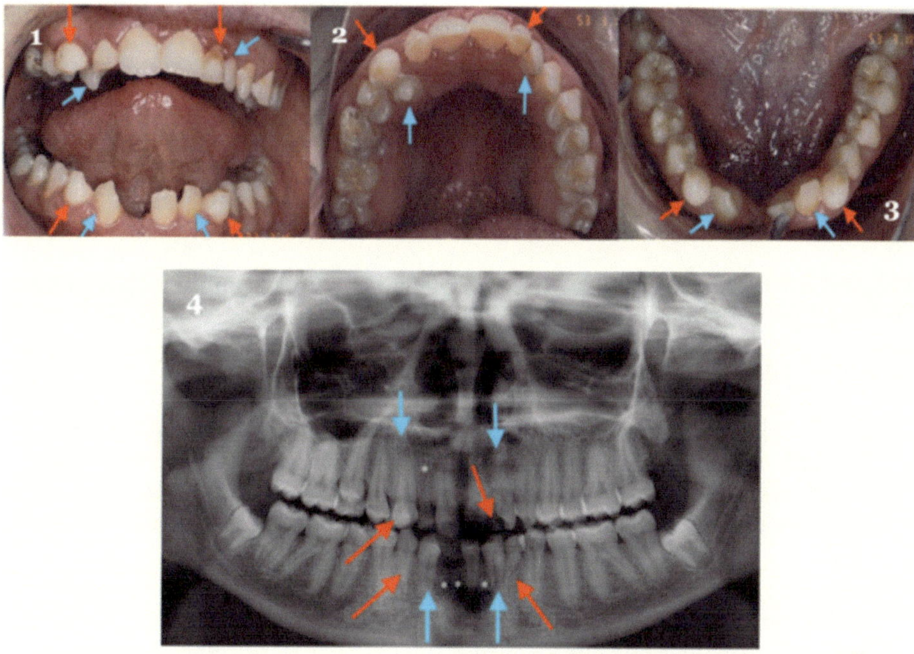

	Right quadrants	Left quadrants
Upper teeth (maxillary)	* 8 7 6 5 4 3 2 1	1 2 3 4 5 6 7 8
Lower teeth (mandibular)	8 7 6 5 4 3 2 1 * *	1 2 3 4 5 6 7 8 *

Figure 7.
*Multiple tooth agenesis in a 14-year-old female patient with trisomy 21. (1–3) intraoral photos reveal a mixed dentition. It is important to note that the prolonged retention of several primary teeth, either due to the congenital absence of the permanent successor tooth (which is the case of the missing maxillary right lateral incisor) or the deviation in the eruptive path of the permanent successor which determinate the concomitant presence of both the deciduous and the permanent teeth on the arch (in the figures, the deciduous teeth are marked with red arrows while the permanent ones are labeled by blue arrows). The degree of complexity involved in this case is increased not only by the agenesis of the upper right lateral incisor, but its association with another three missing incisors in the lower arch. (4) based on the anamnesis and the examination of the panoramic radiograph, it was confirmed the agenesis of the upper right lateral incisor, lower lateral incisors, and the lower right central incisor. Moreover, left second molars in both arches present an elongated pulp chamber and apically displaced furcations, which are specific for the diagnosis of taurodontism. * position of the missing teeth.*

enamel hypoplasia and hypocalcification. Irregular alignment is common as well. Tooth eruption of both deciduous and permanent teeth is delayed in 75% of cases and irregular sequence of eruption is common [60]. DS children with missing teeth have a more obvious tendency in developing a Class III relationship of the jaws than DS children without tooth agenesis. This must be taken into account when treating a DS patient [61].

- Wolf-Hirschhorn syndrome and missing teeth (OMIM 194190)

  The deletion of the distal short arm of human chromosome 4 causes del(4p) syndrome known as Wolf-Hirschhorn syndrome. The critical region is 4p16.3 (WHSCR) and lies approximately 2 Mb from the telomere, so that multiple genes are deleted. Most important genes, playing a major role in early development, are NDS2 (nuclear receptor binding SET domain protein 2), LETM1 (leucine zipper and EF-hand containing transmembrane protein 1), and MSX1 (muscle segment homeo box homolog 1) cause the typical signs and symptoms of this disorder, such as characteristic facial appearance (microcephaly, high forehead, prominent glabella," Greek warrior helmet" facies, broad and/or beaked nose, hypertelorism, short philtrum, micrognathia, downturned corners of the mouth, short upper lip, dysplastic ears, preauricular tags), delayed growth and development, intellectual disability, and seizures. Agenesis of many permanent teeth has been reported [60].

About 10% of the patients have cleft lip and palate, 25% present cleft palate, and 50% with micrognathia and high arched palate.

Although, MSX1 gene is outside the WHSCR, in people with Wolf-Hirschhorn syndrome it is frequently deleted. Previous studies reported the critical role of MSX1 in dental, lip, and palate development [62, 63]. Some people with Wolf-Hirschhorn syndrome present mutations of MSX1 gene. It is expected that deletion of MSX1 gene might disrupt the formation of oral structures in early development, causing missing teeth and other dental abnormalities associated with an opening in the roof of the mouth (cleft palate) and/or a split in the upper lip (cleft lip). Nieminen et al. considered that haploinsufficiency of MSX1 gene is a possible mechanism for selective tooth agenesis 1 but a single copy of the gene is not sufficient to produce the oral cleft phenotype [64].

4.7 Sporadic tooth agenesis

Tooth agenesis cases are either familial or sporadic. Sporadic cases are commonly considered to be nonhereditary, with low risk for relatives or offspring.

By definition, a sporadic disorder arises in the absence of evidence for a heritable or environmental etiology. Affected individuals occur occasionally in families with no reported medical history of tooth agenesis. Consequently, apparently sporadic tooth agenesis may be not inherited from parents but may arise from different aetiologies. Fisher et al. considered that apparently sporadic disorders imply genetic or environmental factors. Sporadic cases can arise from new mutations in germs cells or somatic cells, as well as disorders with an environmental cause [65].

Usually, environmental factors may cause arrested tooth development. Different kinds of trauma in the dental region, such as fractures, surgical procedures on the jaw, and extraction of the preceding primary tooth are mentioned in the literature, as reviewed by Arte [18]. Furthermore, Vastardis H. [46] reported that dental agenesis in association with other developmental abnormalities may occur because of syphilis, scarlet fever, rickets or nutritional disorders during pregnancy or childhood that act in the early stages of a developmental process. Besides, the authors emphasized the effects of cranial irradiation on endocrine function and tooth development.

5. Genetic testing and diagnosis

Tooth agenesis is diagnosed by intraoral examination (teeth did not erupt), radiographic assessment of oral cavity (no visible mineralization), and a detailed dental history to rule out extractions and trauma. Unusual spacing in a child's dentition should lead the parent or dentist to suspect tooth agenesis. Occasionally, tooth agenesis could be a clinical sign of a possible underlying syndrome and not only an isolated disease. Referrals to genetic specialists should be considered if a dentist suspects a patient is affected with tooth agenesis.

Using genetic testing, it is possible to screen or diagnose a patient and make a precise etiological diagnosis. Tooth agenesis may occur without a family history, although it is often familial. Monogenic forms of tooth agenesis have a strong genetic component and genetic testing has usually a confirmatory role. The known mutations in some genes can be screened for early signs of developing problems and identification of the individuals at risk.

The analysis is available for genes involved in both syndromic and non-syndromic forms of tooth agenesis, but the test is expensive, and it is not always covered by health insurance.

Known genotype–phenotype correlations can be used for mutation detection. Clinical features in tooth agenesis might be predictive of underlying genotype. For example, if specific teeth are missing, such as maxillary first premolars associated with MSX1 mutations or lateral incisors associated with WNT10B mutations, tooth agenesis pattern gives clue to the most appropriate genetic tests to follow. Genetic testing panel for selective tooth agenesis analyses changes in nine genes at once. Looking for tooth agenesis-associated gene mutations, MSX1, PAX9, WNT10A, LRP6, EDA, WNT10B cause non-syndromic selective tooth agenesis, AXIN2 causes oligodontia-colorectal cancer syndrome, LTBP3 causes dental anomalies and short stature, and PTH1R causes primary failure of tooth eruption.

http://ctgt.net/panel/oligodontia-selective-tooth-agenesis-ngs-panel

Combining the clinical features with genetic data is possible to increase precision in diagnosis, assess prognosis, and prediction of treatment response, provide information for healthcare management and family planning. Genetic counseling is indicated if an individual has a positive family history. For example, Boogaard et al. [43] consider that by including WNTA10A in the DNA diagnostics of isolated tooth agenesis, the yield of molecular testing in this condition was significantly increased from 15% to 71%.

6. Tooth agenesis associated with other clinical features

Several dental anomalies have been reported in association with congenitally missing teeth. Tooth number reduction is frequently associated with a reduction in tooth size of (microdontia), altered crown morphology (molars with fewer cusps), short-rooted teeth, and enlarged tooth body and pulp chamber (taurodontic molar). The fusion of primary teeth is often followed by hypodontia in the permanent successors.

6.1 Clefting and tooth agenesis

Clefting, or an aberrant space between normally fused tissues, usually occurs as either cleft lip with or without cleft palate (CL/P) or cleft palate only (CPO). Whether cases of clefts with dental anomalies should be considered isolated or syndromic cleft can be debated. However, the co-occurrence of cleft lip/palate and tooth agenesis is sometimes described as CL/P-hypodontia syndrome. Arte [18] described hypodontia as a very common anomaly in patients with oral and facial clefts. More studies analyzed tooth agenesis patterns in unilateral/bilateral, complete/incomplete, CL, CL/P or CPO, inside or outside the cleft region.

Published data show that tooth agenesis is more frequently observed in patients with cleft lip and palate (CLP) or their unaffected sisters and brother than in the general population because of close relationship between tooth and cleft formation with respect to the critical time of development and anatomical position [66–69]. Bartzela et al. reported a higher prevalence of dental anomalies in people with cleft lip and palate than in the non-cleft population, even outside of the cleft region. They studied tooth agenesia patterns in human unilateral and bilateral cleft lip and palate and identified more than 50 different patterns of missing teeth. The most common pattern involved maxillary lateral incisors, and maxillary and mandibular second premolars. The frequency of tooth anomalies seems to be related to the severity of the cleft type. The prevalence of missing teeth reaches 100% in patients with the most severe type of isolated cleft, such as complete bilateral mixed clefting phenotype.

The prevalence of tooth agenesis in people complete unilateral cleft lip and palate has been reported within a range of 48.8% to 75.9% inside the cleft area. The prevalence outside the cleft region was found to be between 27.2% and 48.8% [66]. when compared with the prevalence of tooth agenesis in general population, which ranges between 3.2% to 7.6%, the prevalence of tooth agenesis in non-affected siblings of cleft lip and palate patients was found to be 11.1% outside the cleft area [11, 70].

The high prevalence of missing teeth outside of cleft region suggests the common genetic background for both tooth agenesis and clefts. So, odontogenesis and palate formation are developmentally related events, and one gene or few genes, might be involved in both processes, in common genetic pathways. Other studies reported no absence of permanent teeth in the maxillary arch outside the cleft (distal to the canines) in unoperated patients with cleft, suggesting that the surgical procedure done to close palatal clefts disrupts the formation of the developing tooth buds, as reviewed by Slayton et al [68].

Slayton et al. provided an overview of published data related to similar genetic component for non-syndromic simultaneous presence of both orofacial clefts and hypodontia. The combined phenotype of tooth agenesis with orofacial clefts outside the cleft region was described in both humans and animal models and provide evidence to support a common genetic etiology. Mouse knockout models for deficiency of MSX1 and PAX9 failed to form teeth and had cleft palate [68].

Few monogenic disorders, such as Van der Woude syndrome (caused by mutation in the IRF6 gene - interferon regulatory factor 6), ectrodactyly-ectodermal dysplasia-clefting syndrome 3 (caused by mutation in the TP63 gene - tumor protein p63), and Kallmann's syndrome (caused by mutation in the FGFR1 gene - fibroblast growth factor receptor 1) have both clefting and hypodontia as typical phenotypic findings (**Table A1**). It should be pointed out that the same gene, IRF6 (interferon regulatory factor 6) may cause a disease as rare as Van der Woude syndrome and also to contribute to much more common defects, such as isolated cleft with or without cleft palate [71].

6.2 Disturbances of teeth eruption and tooth agenesis

Primary failure of tooth eruption (OMIM 125350) was reported in association with hypodontia. The most affected teeth are first, and second molars and involvement can be unilateral or bilateral. Based on family studies, the reported pattern of inheritance was consistent with autosomal dominant ones and molecular cause involved mutation of PTHR1 gene (parathyroid hormone 1 receptor) located on 3p21.31 [72]. Regarding permanent dentition, delayed development of posterior permanent teeth in association with the third molar agenesis was reported in the literature, as reviewed by Nieminen [3]. An average delay of two years was observed, with great variation, in a group of 85 patients with agenesis of on the average seven permanent teeth. It was also reported excessive retardation of development of teeth contralateral to missing teeth. Schalk-van der Weide [25] reported a tendency of early developing teeth of males to be retarded in association with severe agenesis, and in females with severe agenesis second mandibular molars to be significantly delayed in development (only mandibular teeth were studied). The delay correlated with the extent of agenesis was most prominent in positions next to the teeth that had failed to develop.

6.3 Reduction in tooth size and shape

In population studies the relationship of tooth agenesis and microdontia has been shown to be statistically significant. Microdont teeth is small enough to be outside the usual limit of variation and along with the reduction in size, these teeth often exhibit a change in shape. Microdont teeth may be either usual form or with tapering (peg or conical) crowns (**Figure 8**). The most common form of microdontia is localized type, affecting maxillary incisors. Peg maxillary lateral incisors are seen in 1.2 to 3.2% of general population. This is a genetic trait which is manifest as either peg or missing maxillary lateral incisors. The microdont teeth show an autosomal dominant inheritance pattern and variable expressivity. Some studies reported families in which both genitors have pegged permanent maxillary lateral incisors. Their children had severe tooth agenesis involving primarily agenesis of succedaneous permanent teeth. It was suggested that children expressed the gene mutation in homozygous status. Some studies reported a 2:1 preference for the left side. In addition, reduced tooth sizes have also been observed within the healthy

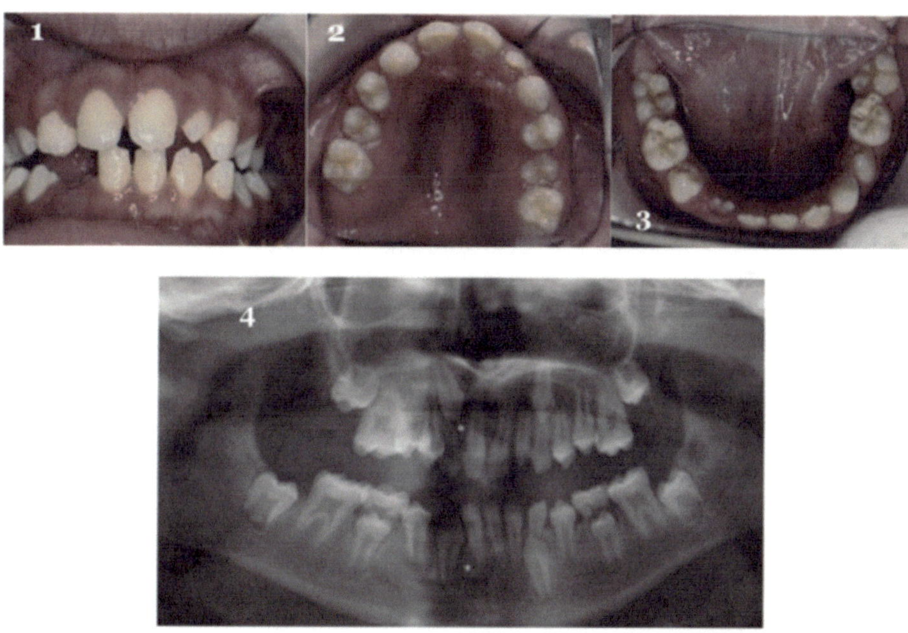

	Right quadrants	Left quadrants
Upper teeth (maxillary)	* 8 7 6 5 4 3 2 1	1 2 3 4 5 6 7 8
Lower teeth (mandibular)	8 7 6 5 4 3 2 1 *	1 2 3 4 5 6 7 8

Figure 8.
*Tooth agenesis in a down syndrome male patient, aged 8 years old. (1–3) intraoral evaluation shows the absence of the right lateral incisors both in the upper and lower arches. (4) the panoramic radiograph confirms the agenesis of maxillary right lateral incisor which is associated to a peg-shaped in the contralateral quadrant. Moreover, agenesis of the lower right lateral incisor is also revealed together with a hypotaurodontism in all four first molars. * position of the missing teeth.*

relatives of patients with severe tooth agenesis [3]. Baccetti [73] reported a significant reciprocal association between agenesis of second premolars and reduced upper lateral incisors. Third molar agenesis was associated with reduction in the cusp number of the molars, as reviewed by Arte [18]. The association of microdontia and tooth agenesis is frequently observed in Down syndrome and various types of ectodermal dysplasia. Generalized microdontia of all teeth is extremely rare in people without some sort of syndrome.

6.4 Malposition of teeth

Abnormal positions, or ectopic placement, of teeth (OMIM 189490) are believed to result from a disturbance of the tooth developmental structure. Various forms of the position or eruption disturbance of teeth tend to be associated with tooth agenesis. Differences in frequencies of the abnormal trait between population groups have been observed, as well as differences in the pattern of associations among displaced maxillary canines (a typical type of malposition of canines) and tooth agenesis.

Pirinen et al. [74] studied the palatal displacement of the canine in regard to congenital absence of permanent teeth in 106 Finnish probands and their first- and second-degree relatives. All the probands had had surgical and orthodontic treatment for displaced maxillary canines. Incisor-premolar hypodontia and peg-shaped incisors were found to be strongly associated with palatally displaced canines. The authors concluded that palatally displaced canine belongs to a spectrum of dental anomalies related to incisor-premolar hypodontia.

Peck et al. reported a strong association of displaced maxillary canines with third molar agenesis and second premolar agenesis, whereas upper lateral incisor agenesis was not significantly interrelated [75]. Garib et al. reported an increased occurrence of displaced maxillary canines associated with second premolars agenesis [76]. Lagana et al. concluded that only the agenesis of maxillary lateral incisors should be considered directly connected with displaced maxillary canine [77].

6.5 Taurodontism

Taurodontism (OMIM 272700) is characterized by large pulp chambers, with changes usually most striking in the molars. The taurodont tooth lies deep in alveolar bone. Taurodont teeth are associated with missing teeth in chromosome aneuploydies, such as Down syndrome (**Figure 9**). It occurs also in other syndromes, especially those having an ectodermal defect, e.g., otodental dysplasia. A family having affected sibs with a combination of sparse hair, oligodontia, and taurodontism was reported in the literature [78].

6.6 Rotation of premolars and/or maxillary lateral incisors

It has been documented by Baccetti T. [73] that rotation of premolars is significantly associated with missing upper lateral incisors. The author found a significant association between unilateral agenesis of upper lateral incisors and rotation of the lateral incisor on the other side of the dental arch, and between unilateral agenesia of premolars and rotation of premolars on the other side of the arch.

6.7 Enamel hypoplasia, hypocalcification

The finding that there is a significant association between enamel hypoplasia and hypodontia not involving systemic syndromes has been reported by Baccetti T. [73]

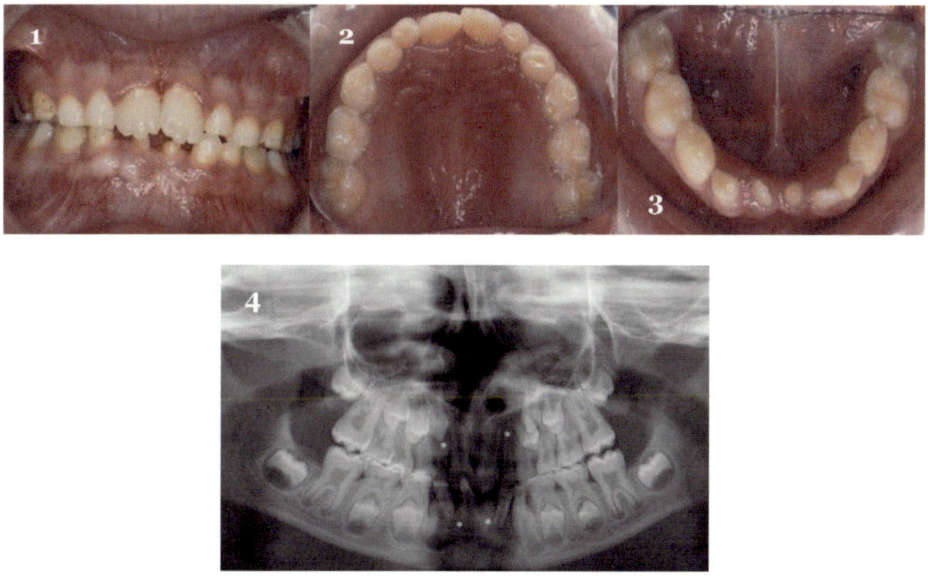

	Right quadrants	Left quadrants
Upper teeth (maxillary)	* 8 7 6 5 4 3 2 1	* 1 2 3 4 5 6 7 8
Lower teeth (mandibular)	8 7 6 5 4 3 2 1 *	1 2 3 4 5 6 7 8 *

Figure 9.
*Multiple tooth agenesis in an 8-year-old male patient with down syndrome. (1,2,3) examination of the dental arches reveals a mixed dentition, with a delayed tooth eruption pattern. (4) panoramic radiograph showing the absence of both the lateral incisors in the maxillary arch and the agenesis of the lower right lateral incisor and the left central incisor. Moreover, the agenesis is associated with mesotaurodont first molars in both upper and lower arches * position of the missing teeth.*

and Lai et al. [79] It may indicate a common genetic origin for both dental anomalies. However, it also is possible that a single or concurrent environmental factor may have been responsible for the etiology of both defects. Some authors have noted that local infection, as well as radiation, may cause both hypodontia and enamel hypoplasia, as review by Lai et al. [79]

6.8 Concomitant hypo-hyperdontia (CHH)

Concomitant hypo-hyperdontia (CHH) is a rare mixed numeric dental anomaly characterized by congenitally missing teeth and supernumerary teeth occurring in the same individual. These two conditions are considered as the opposite extremes in the development of the dentition [80]. The prevalence of CHH was found to range from 0.002 to 0.7%. Due to its rarity and sporadicity, the causes of CHH have been completely unknown. So far, only 80 cases have been reported in the literature. Wang et al. summarized prior research and concluded that more than two-thirds of cases had one supernumerary tooth, and the remaining, two or more teeth. The most commonly supernumerary tooth was mesiodens. Most frequently missing teeth were upper lateral incisors, lower incisors, and premolars. Only a few cases had canines and molars agenesis. Both jaws were affected, bimaxillary hypo-hyperdontia, in about three fourth of the cases. The remaining one-fourth presented maxillary hypo-hyperdontia, the only maxilla being involved [81]. In most cases,

CHH was diagnosed during a regular dental examination. Recently, Wang et al. [81] presented 21 cases of CHH, including 4 familial cases and a syndromic case, and scrutinized their dental phenotypes. Their study results indicated molar taurodontism as the most frequently (29%) observed concurrent dental anomaly of CHH. They also described the fusion of primary lower lateral incisors and canines followed by missing permanent lower laterals. More results described the central cusps of premolars identifiable from the panoramic radiograph of 3 cases. Only one case presented macrodontia of tooth number 9 (upper left central incisor), a premaxillary supernumerary toothand missing tooth number 10 (upper left lateral incisor). The authors concluded," these concurrent dental aberrations suggested that molecular and cellular mechanisms regulating tooth number also play significant roles in tooth morphogenesis".

7. Conclusions

Tooth agenesis has a high prevalence in human population. It was documented that missing tooth has a negative impact on daily quality of life causing significant complications, such as physical appearance problems, oral functional limitations, or psychosocial distress, and cost not only for the affected individual but also for the public health care system worldwide. Early diagnosis is still the best way to prevent complications of missing teeth but understanding the genetic make-up of affected individuals, the dentist must integrate the tools of genetics in the dental practice for prediction, prevention, and personalized dental therapy.

Conflict of interest

The authors declare no conflict of interest.

DOI: http://dx.doi.org/10.5772/intechopen.99419

Appendix 1 – Table A1

Syndrome name and prevalence	Tooth agenesis - levels of severity	Associated phenotypic features by region	Genetic cause	Inheritance	OMIM Orpha-code
ADULT syndrome *acro-dermato-ungual-lacrimal-tooth* <1/1,000,000	**Hypodontia / Oligodontia** associated dental anomalies: small teeth, dysplastic teeth, premature loss of secondary teeth (<25 years)	*Eyes* • Lacrimal duct obstruction • Conjunctivitis *Breasts* • Breast hypoplasia • Mammary gland hypoplasia • Widely spaced nipples • Absent nipples • Hypoplastic nipples *Hands and feet* • Ectrodactyly • Syndactyly *Skin* • Ectodermal dysplasia • Atrophic skin • Thin skin • Dry skin • Freckling • Photosensitive skin • Dermatitis • Adermatoglyphia *Nails* • Dysplastic nails • Nail pits *Hair* • Blond hair • Thin scalp hair • Sparse axillary hair • Premature scalp hair loss (>30 years)	mutations of TP63 gene (tumor protein p63) 3q28	AD	103285 978

Syndrome name and prevalence	Tooth agenesis - levels of severity	Associated phenotypic features by region	Genetic cause	Inheritance	OMIM Orpha-code
Axenfeld-Rieger syndrome, type 1 1/200,000	**Hypodontia** (maxillary incisors)	*Face* • Maxillary hypoplasia • Short philtrum • Prominent supraorbital ridges *Eyes* • Iris dysplasia (goniodysgenesis) • Iris hypoplasia • Prominent Schwalbe line (posterior embryotoxon) • Glaucoma • Displaced pupils • Dyscoria • Polycoria • Aniridia • Microcornea • Megalocornea • Strabismus *Nose* • Broad nasal bridge *Mouth* • Thin upper lip **ABDOMEN** *External Features* • Umbilical defect (redundant periumbilical skin) *Gastrointestinal* • Imperforate anus • Anal stenosis **GENITOURINARY** *External Genitalia (Male)* • Hypospadias	mutations of PITX2 (paired-like homeodomain transcription factor 2) 4q25	AD Genetic heterogeneity Variable expressivity	180500 782

Syndrome name and prevalence	Tooth agenesis - levels of severity	Associated phenotypic features by region	Genetic cause	Inheritance	OMIM Orpha-code
		ENDOCRINE FEATURES • Growth hormone deficiency			
Ectodermal dysplasia 3, Witkop type 1–2/10,000	Normal to small primary teeth Partial to total absence of permanent teeth (**anodontia**)	*Face* • Normal facies *Mouth* • Lip eversion *Skin* • Normal sweat glands *Nails* • Thin, small friable nails • Koilonychia • Longitudinal ridging • Nail pits • Toenails often more affected than fingernails • Nail changes improve with age *Hair* • Normal hair	mutations of MSX1 (muscle segment homeobox 1) 4p16.1	AD	189500 2228
Ectrodactyly, Ectodermal Dysplasia, and cleft lip/palate syndrome 3; EEC type 3 1–9/100.000	**Selective tooth agenesis** Microdontia Caries	*Face* • Maxillary hypoplasia • Malar hypoplasia *Ears* • Hearing loss • Small ears • Malformed auricles *Eyes* • Blue irides • Photophobia • Blepharophimosis • Blepharitis • Dacryocystitis	mutations of TP63 *(tumor protein p73-like; tp73l p53-related protein p63)* 3q28	AD	604292 1896

Syndrome name and prevalence	Tooth agenesis - levels of severity	Associated phenotypic features by region	Genetic cause	Inheritance	OMIM Orpha-code
		• Lacrimal duct abnormalities *Nose* • Flat nasal tip *Mouth* • Cleft lip • Cleft palate • Xerostomia • Absence of Stensen duct **ENDOCRINE FEATURES** • Growth hormone deficiency • Hypogonadotropic hypogonadism • Central diabetes insipidus			
Hypohidrotic ectodermal dysplasia 1 (XHED) or Christ-Siemens-Touraine syndrome 1/15,000 (1/50,000 to 1/100,000 male births)	**Hypodontia** **Adontia** Microdontia Conical teeth Taurodontism	*Head* • Small cranial length *Face* • Frontal bossing • Hypoplastic maxilla • Small chin • Small facial height • Prominent supraorbital ridges *Eyes* • Periorbital wrinkles • Periorbital hyperpigmentation • Absent tears • Absent miebomian glands • Scant-absent eyebrows • Scant-absent eyelashes *Nose* • Small nose • Hypoplastic alae nasi • Nasal mucosa atrophy	mutations of EDA (ectrodysplasin A) Xq13.1	X-linked recessive Xq13.1 Heterozygous females show variable expressivity (mild to severe manifestations) including hypodontia, conical teeth, reduction in scalp/body hair, and difficulty nursing	305100 238468

Syndrome name and prevalence	Tooth agenesis - levels of severity	Associated phenotypic features by region	Genetic cause	Inheritance	OMIM Orpha-code
		• Ozena • Depressed nasal root and bridge ('saddle nose') *Mouth* • Decreased palatal depth • Prominent lips **RESPIRATORY** • Respiratory difficulties *Nasopharynx* • Atrophic rhinitis • Atrophic pharyngeal mucosa • Hypoplastic or absent mucous glands which may lead to dried secretions and obstruction *Larynx* • Atrophic mucosa causing dysphonia **CHEST** *Breasts* • Hypoplastic-absent mammary glands • Hypoplastic-absent nipples **SKIN, NAILS, & HAIR** *Skin* • Hypohidrosis • Anhidrosis • Sweat pore aplasia • Soft, thin skin • Dry skin • Mild localized pigmentation abnormalities • Skin peeling/scaling (newborn)			

Syndrome name and prevalence	**Tooth agenesis - levels of severity**	**Associated phenotypic features by region**	**Genetic cause**	**Inheritance**	**OMIM Orpha-code**
		• Eczema • Periorbital wrinkling • Periorbital hyperpigmentation • Hypoplastic-absent sebaceous glands • Hypoplastic-absent eccrine sweat glands *Nails* • Spoon-shaped nails *Hair* • Hypotrichosis • Fine, brittle hair • Scanty hair • Absent or scanty eyelashes • Absent or scanty eyebrows • Blonde, fine scalp hair **VOICE** • Hoarse voice due to dry laryngeal mucosa **METABOLIC FEATURES** • Intolerance to heat and fevers • Susceptible to hyperthermia			
Kallmann syndrome 2 hypogonado-tropic hypogonadism 2 with or without anosmia; HH2 1/8,000 males and 1/40,000 females, but is probably underestimated.	**Tooth agenesis, variable in number** (in some patients)	**HEAD & NECK** *Ears* • Hearing loss, unilateral (rare) *Eyes* • Iris coloboma (rare) *Nose* • Hyposmia/anosmia (in some patients) • Absence of nasal cartilage, unilateral (rare)	mutation of FGFR1 (fibroblast growth factor receptor 1) 8p11.23	AD	147950 478

Syndrome name and prevalence	Tooth agenesis - levels of severity	Associated phenotypic features by region	Genetic cause	Inheritance	OMIM Orpha-code
		Mouth • Cleft lip • Cleft palate **SKELETAL** • Osteopenia (in some patients) *Hands* • Clinodactyly (rare) • Fusion of fourth and fifth metacarpal bones (rare) • Ectrodactyly (rare) *Feet* • Ectrodactyly (rare) **ENDOCRINE FEATURES** • Hypogonadotropic hypogonadism • Delayed or absent puberty • Low to undetectable gonadotropin levels • Low testosterone level • Low estradiol level **GENITOURINARY** *External Genitalia (Male)* • Micropenis • Cryptorchidism *Internal Genitalia (Female)* • Primary amenorrhea			
KBG syndrome *macrodontia, mental retardation, characteristic facies, short stature, and skeletal anomalies* unkown prevalence	**Oligodontia** Associated dental anomalies: macrodontia of the upper central incisors, wide upper central incisors, ridged teeth, fused incisors	*head* • microcephaly *face* • round face early in life • triangular face later in life • long philtrum	ankrd11 (ankyrin repeat-containing cofactor 1) 16q24.3	AD	148050 2332

Syndrome name and prevalence	Tooth agenesis - levels of severity	Associated phenotypic features by region	Genetic cause	Inheritance	OMIM Orpha-code
		ears • large prominent ears *eyes* • hypertelorism • telecanthus • long palpebral fissures • broad bushy eyebrows *nose* • anteverted nares • hypoplastic alae nasi **chest** *ribs sternum clavicles & scapulae* • cervical rib fusion • accessory cervical ribs **genitourinary** *internal genitalia (male)* • cryptorchidism **skeletal** • delayed bone maturation *spine* • vertebral body fusion • vertebral arch abnormalities • thoracic kyphosis *hands* • clinodactyly • decreased hand length • syndactyly **skin, nails, & hair** *skin* • simian crease *hair* • broad bushy eyebrows			

DOI: http://dx.doi.org/10.5772/intechopen.99419

Syndrome name and prevalence	Tooth agenesis - levels of severity	Associated phenotypic features by region	Genetic cause	Inheritance	OMIM Orpha-code
		• low anterior hairline • low posterior hairline **neurologic** *central nervous system* • developmental delay • mental retardation • eeg anomalies (in some patients) • seizures (in some patients)			
Oral-facial-digital syndrome, type 1 (OFD1) 1/50,000 – 1/250,000	Dental caries Anomalous anterior teeth Enamel hypoplasia Supernumerary teeth **Missing teeth**	*Head* • Microcephaly *Face* • Frontal bossing • Facial asymmetry • Microretrognathia • Hypoplasia of the malar bones *Ears* • Low-set ears • Hearing loss *Eyes* • Epicanthus • Hypertelorism • Telecanthus • Downslanting palpebral fissures *Nose* • Broad nasal bridge • Hypoplastic alar cartilage *Mouth* • Hyperplastic oral frenuli • Buccal frenuli • Median cleft lip (in 45% of patients)	mutations of OFD1 gene Xp22.2	X-linked DOMINANT Xp22.2 (usually lethal in males)	311200 2750

Syndrome name and prevalence	Tooth agenesis - levels of severity	Associated phenotypic features by region	Genetic cause	Inheritance	OMIM Orpha-code
		• Pseudocleft of the upper lip • Lobulated tongue (30–45%) • Bifid tongue (30–45%) • Tongue nodule • Cleft palate • Tongue hamartoma (70%) • High-arched palate • Thickened alveolar ridges • Irregular margin of the lips **CARDIOVASCULAR** *Heart* • Cardiac anomalies **ABDOMEN** *Liver* • Fibrocystic liver (45%) • Dilatation and beading of the intrahepatic bile ducts • Hepatic fibrosis *Pancreas* • Pancreatic cysts (29%) **GENITOURINARY** *Internal Genitalia (Female)* • Ovarian cysts *Kidneys* • Adult onset polycystic kidney (50%) **SKELETAL** *Hands* • Abnormalities of the fingers (45%) • Clinodactyly • Syndactyly • Brachydactyly			

Syndrome name and prevalence	Tooth agenesis - levels of severity	Associated phenotypic features by region	Genetic cause	Inheritance	OMIM Orpha-code
		• Polydactyly, preaxial or postaxial (rare) • X-ray shows irregular pattern of radiolucency and/or spicule-like formation in metacarpals and phalanges *Feet* • Abnormalities of the toes (25%) • Duplication of the hallux • Polydactyly, preaxial or postaxial (rare) **SKIN, NAILS, & HAIR** *Skin* • Milia of upper face and ears (infancy) • Dry scalp *Hair* • Dry, rough, sparse hair • Alopecia **NEUROLOGIC** *Central Nervous System* • Variable mental retardation (40%) • Central nervous system malformations (40%) • Abnormal gyrations • Absence of corpus callosum • Gray matter heterotopias • Myelomeningocele (rare) • Stenosis of the aqueduct of Sylvius (rare) • Hydrocephalus • Arachnoid cysts			

Syndrome name and prevalence	**Tooth agenesis - levels of severity**	**Associated phenotypic features by region**	**Genetic cause**	**Inheritance**	**OMIM Orpha-code**
		• Cerebellar abnormalities • Seizures • Hypothalamic hamartoma • Porencephaly *Behavioral Psychiatric Manifestations* • Major depression (rare) **LABORATORY ABNORMALITIES** • Abnormal liver enzymes in those with hepatic cysts or fibrosis • Proteinuria in those with cystic kidneys			
Van der Woude syndrome 1 (VWS1) 1/35,000 – 1/100,000	**Hypodontia**	*Mouth* • Lower lip pits • Cleft lip • Cleft palate • Cleft uvula	mutations of IRF6 gene (interferon regulatory factor 6) 1q32.2	AD	119300 888

Table A1.
Tooth agenesis associated frequent in genetic syndromes based on OMIM database.

Author details

Emilia Severin[1*], George Gabriel Moldoveanu[2] and Andreea Moldoveanu[3]

1 Genetics Department, Carol Davila University of Medicine and Pharmacy, Bucharest, Romania

2 Department of Anaesthesiology and Intensive Care, C.I. Parhon National Institute of Endocrinology, Bucharest, Romania

3 Department of Preventive Dentistry, Carol Davila University of Medicine and Pharmacy, Bucharest, Romania

*Address all correspondence to: emilia.severin@umfcd.ro

References

[1] Congenital anomalies [website]. Geneva: World Health Organization; 2020 Avaiable from: (http://www.who.int/mediacentre/factsheets/fs370/en/index.htmlexternal icon [Accessed 2020 Decembre 2020]

[2] Ohazama A, and Sharpe PT. 2008. Development of Epidermal Appendages: Teeth and Hair in Inborn Errors of Development, edited by Epstein CJ, Erickson RP, Wynshaw-Boris A, 2nd Edition, Oxford University Press. 245-251.

[3] Nieminen P. Molecular Genetics of Tooth Agenesis, Academic Dissertation, Helsinki 2007;39-40.

[4] Vastardis H, Karimbux N, Guthua SW, Seidman JG, and Seidman CE. 1996. A human MSX1 homeodomain missense mutation causes selective tooth agenesis. Nat Genet 13: 417-421.

[5] OMIM: Avaiable from: https://www.omim.org/entry/106600?search=hypodontia&highlight=hypodontia, [Accessed 2020 Decembre 25]

[6] Arte S, Nieminen P, Apajalahti S, Haavikko K, Thesleff I, and Pirinen S. 2001a. Characteristics of incisor-premolar hypodontia in families. J Dent Res, 80, 1445-1450.

[7] Mattheeuws N, Dermaut L, Martens G. Has hypodontia increased in Caucasians during the 20th century? A meta-analysis. Eur J Orthod. 2004;26: 99–103.

[8] Nieminen P. 2009. Genetic basis of tooth agenesis. J Exp Zool B Mol Dev Evol. 312B(4):320-342.

[9] Yonezu T., Hayashi Y., Sasaki J., Machida Y. Prevalence of congenital dental anomalies of the deciduous dentition in Japanese children. The Bulletin of Tokyo Dental College. 1997; 38(1):27–32.

[10] Matalova E, Fleischmannova J, Sharpe PT, Tucker AS. 2008. Tooth agenesis: From molecular genetics to molecular dentistry. J Dent Res. 87(7): 617-623.

[11] Polder BJ, Van't Hof MA, Van der Linden FPGM, Kuijpers-Jagtman AM. A meta-analysis of the prevalence of dental agenesis of permanent teeth. Community Dent Oral Epidemiol. 2004; 32:217–226.

[12] Larmour CJ, Mossey PA, Thind BS, Forgie AH, Stirrups DR. Hypodontia - a retrospective review of prevalence and etiology. Part I. Quintessence Int. 2005; 36:263–270.

[13] Shimizu T, Maeda T. Prevalence and genetic basis of tooth agenesis. Japanese Dental Science Review. 2009;45:52–58.

[14] Rakhshan V. Congenitally missing teeth (hypodontia): A review of the literature concerning the etiology, prevalence, risk factors, patterns and treatment. Dent Res J (Isfahan). 2015; 12(1):1-13. doi:10.4103/1735-3327.150286

[15] Rakhshan V. Meta-analysis and systemic review of factors biasing the observed prevalence of congenitally missing teeth in permanent dentition excluding third molars. Prog Orthod. 2013;14:33.

[16] Shetty P, Adyanthaya A, Adyanthaya S, Sreelatha SV. The prevalence of hypodontia and supernumerary teeth in 2469 school children of the Indian population: An epidemiological study. Indian J Stomatol. 2012;3:150–152.

[17] Gábris K, Tarján I, Csiki P, Konrád F, Szádeczky B, Rózsa N. A

maradó fogak csírahiányának elófordulási gyakorisága és a kezelés lehetóségei [Prevalence of congenital hypodontia in the permanent dentition and its treatment]. Fogorv Sz. 2001 Aug; 94(4):137–40. Hungarian. PMID: 11573454.

[18] Arte S. Phenotypic and Genotypic Features of Familial Hypodontia. Academic Disertation, Helsinki, Finland, 2001, 14-21.

[19] Gracco ALT, Zanatta S, Valvecchi F, *et al.* Prevalence of dental agenesis in a sample of Italian orthodontic patients: an epidemiological study. Prog Orthod. 18, 33 (2017). https://doi.org/10.1186/s40510-017-0186-9

[20] Gomes RR, da Fonseca JA, Paula LM, Faber J, Acevedo AC. Prevalence of hypodontia in orthodontic patients in Brasilia, Brazil. Eur J Orthod 2010;32:302-306.

[21] Eshgian N et al., Prevalence of hyperdontia, hypodontia, and concomitant hypo-hyperdontia, Journal of Dental Sciences, 2021, Volume 16, Issue 2:713-717. https://doi.org/10.1016/j.jds.2020.09.005

[22] Rakhshan V, Rakhshan H. Meta-analysis of congenitally missing teeth in the permanent dentition: Prevalence, variations across ethnicities, regions and time. Int Orthod. 2015 Sep;13(3):261–73. English, French. doi: 10.1016/j.ortho.2015.06.008. Epub 2015 Aug 14. PMID: 26279516.

[23] Pemberton TJ, Das P and Patel PI, Hypodontia: Genetics and future perspectives. Brazilian Journal of Oral Science, 2005; 4:695-706.

[24] Fekonja A. Hypodontia in orthodontically treated children. Eur J Orthod. 2005 Oct;27(5):457-460. doi: 10.1093/ejo/cji027. Epub 2005 Jul 25. PMID: 16043466.

[25] Schalk-van der Weide Y, Steen WHA, Bosman F, Distribution of missing teeth and tooth morphology in patients with oligodontia, J Dent Child 1992; 59: 133-140.

[26] Rolling S, Poulsen S. Oligodontia in Danish schoolchildren. Acta Odontol Scand 2001; 59: 111-2.26

[27] Daugaard-Jensen J, Nodal M, Skovgaard LT, Kjaer I. Comparison of the pattern of agenesis in the primary and permanent dentitions in a population characterized by agenesis in the primary dentition. International Journal of Paediatric Dentistry, 1997; 7: 143–148.

[28] Harris EF, Clark LL. Hypodontia: an epidemiologic study of American black and white people. Am J Orthod Dentofacial Orthop. 2008;134(6): 761–767. 10.1016/j.ajodo.2006.12.019

[29] Lee SH, Lee JY, Park HK, Kim YK. Development of third molars in Korean juveniles and adolescents. Forensic Sci Int. 2009;188(1–3): 107–111. 10.1016/j.forsciint.2009.03.033

[30] Davis PJ. **Hypodontia and hyperdontia of permanent teeth in Hong Kong children**. Community Dent Oral Epidemiol,1987, 15, pp. 218-220

[31] Thesleff I. Two genes for missing teeth. Nature Genetics,1996, 13: 379–380.

[32] Pinho T, Tavares P, Maciel P, Pollmann C. Developmental absence of maxillary lateral incisors in the Portuguese population. Eur J Orthod. 2005;27(5):443–449.

[33] Juuri E, Balic A. The biology underlying abnormalities of tooth number in humans. J Dent Res. 2017;96 (11):1248–1256.

[34] Goya HA, Tanaka S, Maeda T, Akimoto Y. An orthopantomographic

study of hypodontia in permanent teeth of Japanese pediatric patients. J Oral Sci 2008;50:143-150.

[35] Kirzioglu Z, Sentut TK, Erturk MSO, Karayilmaz H. Clinical features of hypodontia and associated dental anomalies: a retrospective study. Oral Dis. 2005;11(6):399–404.

[36] Endo T, Ozoe R, Kubota M, Akiyama M, Shimooka S. A survey of hypodontia in Japanese orthodontic patients.Am J Orthod Dentofac Orthop. 2006;129:29

[37] Chung CJ, Han JH, Kim KH. The pattern and prevalence of hypodontia in Koreans. Oral Dis. 2008 Oct;14(7): 620-625. doi: 10.1111/ j.1601-0825.2007.01434.x. Epub 2008 Feb 1. PMID: 18248591.

[38] Medina AC. Radiographic study of prevalence and distribution of hypodontia in a pediatric orthodontic population in Venezuela. Pediatr Dent 2012;34:113-116.

[39] Pirinen S, Thesleff I. Development of the dentition. In : Thilander B, Ronning O (eds). Introduction to Orthodontics. Stockholm: Lic Forlag; 1995. p.41-43.

[40] Fournier BP, Bruneau MH, Toupenay S, Kerner S, Berdal A, Cormier-Daire V, Hadj-Rabia S, Coudert AE, de La Dure-Molla M. Patterns of Dental Agenesis Highlight the Nature of the Causative Mutated Genes. J Dent Res. 2018 Nov;97(12): 1306-1316. doi: 10.1177/ 0022034518777460. Epub 2018 Jun 7. PMID: 29879364.

[41] Azza Husam Al-Ani, Joseph Safwat Antoun, William Murray Thomson, Tony Raymond Merriman, Mauro Farella, "Hypodontia: An Update on Its Etiology, Classification, and Clinical Management", BioMedResearch International, vol. 2017, Article ID 9378325, 9 pages, 2017. https://doi.org/ 10.1155/2017/9378325

[42] Liu H, Ding T, Zhan Y, Feng H. A Novel AXIN2 Missense Mutation Is Associated with Non-Syndromic Oligodontia. PLoS One. 2015;10(9): e0138221. doi:10.1371/journal. pone.0138221

[43] van den Boogaard, M-J, Creton, M, Bronkhorst, Y, van der Hout, A, Hennekam, E, Lindhout, D, Cune, M, Ploos van Amstel, HK. **Mutations in WNT10A are present in more than half of isolated hypodontia cases.** J. Med. Genet. 49: 327-331, 2012.

[44] Arte S, Parmanen S, Pirinen S, Alaluusua S, Nieminen P. Candidate gene analysis of tooth agenesis identifies novel mutations in six genes and suggests significant role for WNT and EDA signaling and allele combinations. PLoS One. 2013;8(8):e73705. doi: 10.1371/journal.pone.0073705

[45] Michon F.Tooth evolution and dental defects: from genetic regulation network to micro-RNA fine-tuning. Birth Defects Research. Part A, Clinical and Molecular Teratology.2011.91:763–769.

[46] Vastardis H. The genetics of human tooth agenesis: New discoveries for understanding dental anomalies. American Journal of Orthodontics and Dentofacial Orthopedics. 2000. Volume 117, Number 6. doi.10.1067/ mod.2000.103257

[47] Mostowska A, Biedziak B, Trzeciak W H.A novel c.581C>T transition localized in a highly conserved homeobox sequence of MSX1: is it responsible for oligodontia?.2006 Journal of Applied Genetics.47: 159-164

[48] Townsend G, Hughes T, Luciano M, Bockmann M, Brook A. Genetic and environmental influences on human dental variation: a critical evaluation of

studies involving twins. Arch Oral Biol. 2009;54 Suppl 1(Suppl 1):S45-S51. doi: 10.1016/j.archoralbio.2008.06.009

[49] Dreesen K, Swinnen S, Devriendt K, Carels C. Tooth agenesis patterns and phenotype variation in a cohort of Belgian patients with hypodontia and oligodontia clustered in 79 families with their pedigrees, European Journal of Orthodontics, Volume 36, Issue 1, February 2014, Pages 99–106, https://doi.org/10.1093/ejo/cjt021

[50] Ahmad, W, Brancolini, V, Faiyaz ul Haque, M, Lam, H, ul Haque, S, Haider, M, Maimon, A, Aita, V. M, Owen, J, Brown, D, Zegarelli, D J, Ahmad, M, Ott, J, Christiano, A M. **A locus for autosomal recessive hypodontia with associated dental anomalies maps to chromosome 16q12.1.(Letter)** Am. J. Hum. Genet. 62: 987-991, 1998. PubMed: 9529357.

[51] Wang, H., Zhao, S., Zhao, W., Feng, G., Jiang, S., Liu, W., Li, S., Xue, H., He, L. **Congenital absence of permanent teeth in a six-generation Chinese kindred.** Am. J. Med. Genet. 90: 193-198, 2000. PubMed: 10678655

[52] Huckert, M., Stoetzel, C., Morkmued, S., Laugel-Haushalter, V., Geoffroy, V., Muller, J., Clauss, F., Prasad, M. K., Obry, F., Raymond, J. L., Switala, M., Alembik, Y., and 24 others. Mutations in the latent TGF-beta binding protein 3 (LTBP3) gene cause brachyolmia with amelogenesis imperfecta. Hum. Molec. Genet. 24: 3038-3049, 2015. PubMed: 25669657

[53] Kim, J-W, Simmer, J P, Lin, B P-J, Hu, J C-C. Novel MSX1 frameshift causes autosomal-dominant oligodontia. J. Dent. Res. 2006;85: 267-271.

[54] Yu P, Yang W, Han D, et al. Mutations in WNT10B Are Identified in Individuals with Oligodontia. Am J Hum Genet. 2016;99(1):195-201. doi:10.1016/j.ajhg.2016.05.012

[55] Luder, Hans Ulrich; and Mitsiadis, Thimios A (February 2012) Tooth Agenesis. In: eLS. John Wiley & Sons, Ltd: Chichester. DOI: 10.1002/9780470015902.a0005990.pub2

[56] Townsend G,Bockmann M, Hughes T, Brook A. Genetic, environmental and epigenetic influences on variation in human tooth number, size and shape.2012. Odontology.100:1–9

[57] Gorlin, RJ, Herman, NG, Moss, SJ. **Complete absence of the permanent dentition: an autosomal recessive disorder. (Letter)** Am. J. Med. Genet. 5: 207-209, 1980. PubMed: 7395912

[58] Stranecky, V., Hoischen, A., Hartmannova, H., Zaki, M. S., Chaudhary, A., Zudaire, E., Noskova, L., Baresova, V., Pristoupilova, A., Hodanova, K., Sovova, J., Hulkova, H., and 13 others. **Mutations in ANTXR1 cause GAPO syndrome.** Am. J. Hum. Genet. 92: 792-799, 2013. PubMed: 23602711

[59] Severin E, Paun A, Baltag R, Stan A, Funieru C. Common, rare, and individual oro-dental findings in people with Down syndrome. J Int Oral Health 2016; 8:964–968.

[60] Hennekam RCM, Krantz ID, Allanson JE. Gorlin's Syndrome of the Head and Neck – Chromosomal Syndromes: Common and Well-Known Syndromes. Oxford University Press, 5th Edition.2010.53 and 63.

[61] van Marrewijk DJF, van Stiphout MAE, Reuland-Bosma W, Bronkhorst EM, Ongkosuwito EM, The relationship between craniofacial development and hypodontia in patients with Down syndrome, European Journal of Orthodontics, Volume 38, Issue 2, April 2016, Pages 178–183.

[62] van den Boogaard MJ, Dorland M, Beemer FA, van Amstel HK. MSX1

mutation is associated with orofacial clefting and tooth agenesis in humans. Nat Genet 2000; 24: 342– 343.

[63] Vieira AR, McHenry TG, Daack-Hirsch S, Murray JC, Marazita ML. Candidate gene/loci studies in cleft lip/palate and dental anomalies finds novel susceptibility genes for clefts. Genet Med 2008; 10: 668–674.

[64] Nieminen P, Kotilainen J, Aalto Y, Knuutila S, Pirinen S, Thesleff I. MSX1 gene is deleted in Wolf-Hirschhorn syndrome patients with oligodontia. J Dent Res. 2003 Dec;82(12):1013-1017.

[65] Fisher EM, Lana-Elola E, Watson SD, Vassiliou G, Tybulewicz VL. New approaches for modelling sporadic genetic disease in the mouse. Dis Model Mech. 2009;2(9–10):446-453. doi:10.1242/dmm.001644

[66] Bartzela TN, Carels CEL, Bronkhorst EM, Rønning E, Rizell S, Kuijpers-Jagtman AM. Tooth agenesis patterns in bilateral cleft lip and palate. Eur J Oral Sci 2010; 118: 47–52.

[67] Bartzela TN, Carels CEL, Bronkhorst EM, Kuijpers- Jagtman AM, Tooth agenesis patterns in unilateral cleft lip and palate in humans.Archives of Oral Biology.2013.Volume 58, Issue 6: 596-602.

[68] Slayton RL, Williams L, Murray JC, Wheeler JJ, Lidral AC, Nishimura CJ. Genetic association studies of cleft lip and/or palate with hypodontia outside the cleft region. Cleft Palate Craniofac J. 2003;40(3):274-279. doi:10.1597/1545-1569_2003_040_0274_gasocl_2.0.co_2

[69] Dewinter G, Quirynen M, Heidbuchel K, Verdonck A, Willems G, Carels C. Dental abnormalities, bone graft quality, and periodontal conditions in patients with unilateral cleft lip and palate at different phases of orthodontic treatment Cleft Palate-Craniofacial Journal, 40 (4) (2003), pp. 343-350

[70] Eerens K, Vlietinck R, Heidbuchel K, Van Olmen A, Derom C, Willems G, *et al.* Hypodontia and tooth formation in groups of children with cleft, siblings without cleft, and nonrelated controlsCleft Palate-Craniofacial Journal, 38 (4) (2001), pp. 374-378

[71] Vieira, A. R., et al. Interferon regulatory factor 6 (IRF6) and fibroblast growth factor receptor 1 (FGFR1) contribute to human tooth agenesis. American Journal of Medical Genetics, 2007, 143, 538–545.

[72] Decker E, Stellzig-Eisenhauer A, Fiebig B S, Rau C, Kress W, Saar K, Ruschendorf F, Hubner N, Grimm T, Weber BHF. **PTHR1 loss-of-function mutations in familial, nonsyndromic primary failure of tooth eruption.** Am. J. Hum. Genet. 83: 781-786, 2008. PubMed: 19061984.

[73] Baccetti T. A controlled study of associated dental anomalies. Angle Orthod. 1998.Jun;68(3):267-74. doi: 10.1043/00033219(1998)068<0267: ACSOAD>2.3.CO;2. PMID: 9622764.

[74] Pirinen S, Arte S, Apajalahti S. **Palatal displacement of canine is genetic and related to congenital absence of teeth.** J. Dent. Res. 75: 1742-1746, 1996. PubMed: 8955668

[75] Peck S, Peck L, Kataja M. Prevalence of tooth agenesis and peg-shaped maxillary lateral incisor associated with palatally displaced canine (PDC) anomaly. Am J Orthod Dentofac Orthop. 1996;110:441–443.

[76] Garib DG, Alencar BM, Lauris JR, Baccetti T. Agenesis of maxillary lateral incisors and associated dental anomalies. Am J Orthod Dentofac Orthop. 2010;137(6):732.e1–6.

[77] Laganà G, Venza N,Lione R, Chiaramonte C, Danesi C, Cozza P. Associations between tooth agenesis and

displaced maxillary canines: a cross-sectional radiographic study. Prog Orthod. 2018; 19: 23.

[78] Haunfelder, D. Ein Beitrag zu den Molaren mit prismatischen Wurzel (sog. Taurodontismus). Dtsch. Zahnaerztl. Z. 21: 419-423, 1967.

[79] Lai PY, Seow WK. A controlled study of the association of various dental anomalies with hypodontia of permanent teeth. Pediatr Dent. 1989; 11: 291–296. PubMed

[80] Mallineni SK, Nuvvula S, Cheung AC, Kunduru R. **A comprehensive review of the literature and data analysis on hypo-hyperdontia.** J Oral Sci, 56 (2014), pp. 295-302

[81] Wang YL, Pan HH, Chang HH, Huang GF. Concomitant hypo-hyperdontia: A rare entity. J Dent Sci. 2018;13(1):60-67. doi:10.1016/j.jds.2018.01.001

Chapter 5

Influence of Elements on Gene Expression in Human Teeth

Sukumar Athimoolam

Abstract

Several elements (Ca, Fe, Sr, Mn, Mg, P, Zn, Se, B, Pb, Ni, Ti, etc.), classified mainly under three groups namely beneficial, harmless and harmful elements, are measured in human teeth for multiple purposes since they involve in metabolic activities as well as influence gene expression. There are sufficiently available studies reporting roles of the elements in both up and down-regulation of gene expression leading to tooth repair, regeneration, differentiation, biomineralization and demineralization in the dental stem cells. Considering the importance of tooth developmental and protective roles, the association of the elements with gene expression presented in the present review may facilitate for improvement of their selection as one of the criteria for strengthening teeth for a longer life through nutritional sources and dental material formulation.

Keywords: gene expression, elements, mineralization, demineralization, dental stem cells

1. Introduction

1.1 Inorganic and organic composition

Teeth have major parts of enamel, dentin-pulp complex, and cementum. Dentin, the largest tooth portion, contains a majority of 70% minerals by weight, 20% organic content of the matrix and 10% water [1]. The chief constituent of the organic part of dentine is type I collagen with >85% and collagen types III and V are the other remaining contents of it [2, 3]. The dentine phosphoprotein with ~50% of the noncollagenous part is the main composition of the organic matrix, while hydroxyapatite is found as the remaining composition of inorganic matrix [4, 5]. In the case of enamel, less collagen and more noncollagenous protein of 90% amelogenin were found. The inorganic constituent of these hard tissues is composed of biological apatite, $Ca_{10}(PO_4)_6(OH)_2$. Enamel contains greater inorganic component (~90% prismatic crystals) than dentin (~70%) and cementum (45%) [6]. When the higher inorganic level found is related to higher strength and resistant force in the enamel than in any other hard tissues of body, there are certain means of causing changes in amount of the inorganic constituents linked with both strengthening and weakening of tooth development and structure.

1.2 Element and gene relationship

When essential, non-essential (harmless) and harmful elements reach the dental tissues via blood circulation from natural sources of food, and other man-made sources from environment and dental products used for treatment, the reactions of the tissues rely upon dosage and chemical and biological features of the elements and are markers of specifying the element nature under beneficial, harmful and neutral roles in elucidating actions of gene expression [7, 8]. Since the dental tissues are exposed continuously to multi-elements at varying quantities and with different physiological functions, it is conspicuous to discuss here in details about the consequence of element intake in particular, the interaction between elements and genes. The processes of mineralization and demineralization are important functions of the tissues of teeth and bone and are under the control of several genes identified with varying levels of expression through protein secretion [9]. The diverse genes, levels of expression and related proteins responsible for either strengthening through mineralization and remineralization or debilitating the teeth via demineralization are described well in this review.

1.3 Utilities of dental pulp stem cells

Stem cells are pluripotent cells, having the property of differentiating into various types of cells of the human body [10]. Mesenchymal stem cells (MSCs) that have been developed from various human tissues, peripheral blood and body fluids, are characterized by cellular and molecular markers to understand their specific phenotypes [11]. Dental pulp stem cells (DPSCs) having an MSCs phenotype, can be obtained from different dental tissues viz., human exfoliated deciduous teeth, apical papilla, periodontal ligament (PDL) and dental follicle tissue and can also be developed into induced pluripotent stem cells by incorporation of pluripotency markers [12]. The stem cells isolated from different dental tissues are utilized for in vitro studies about the interaction between elements and gene resulting in gene expression and mineralization. In this chapter, an attempt has been made to explore the relationship of element effects on gene expression in the DPSCs with mineralization, cell differentiation and development of teeth.

2. Influence of genes and mineralization

2.1 Mineralization

The bone, dentin and cementum are the hard connective tissues which under normal biological processes are formed of the collagen fibrils through a scaffold of extremely arranged crystal structures of calcium phosphate [6]. The cells of the hard connective tissues influence various mineralization activities such as crystal structural morphology, composition and localized development and growth. In the bone and the tooth dentin and enamel, the mineral salts of calcium and phosphate ions are fixed through activities of the constituents of the extracellular matrix and a sequence of biocatalysts of enzymes. Mineralization, a lifetime function, occurs through the precipitation of inorganic elements within the matrix of organic components of teeth and bones [13]. Tooth mineralisation processes are implicated with tissues interactions between ectodermal and mesenchymal layers [14] and also with extracellular matrix components and cell-derived microstructures [15]. Knowledge about the mechanism of mineral deposition is essential for prophylaxis and treatments of ill health related to mineralization and also for the renovation and reconstruction of scaffolds.

2.2 Chromosomal defect and mineralization

Alvesalo [16] reported that the Y chromosome regulates the growth of both tooth enamel and dentin, but the X chromosome influences enamel formation only. Hence, various sex chromosome anomalies are associated with variation in tooth crown size and structure of individuals [16] and also with impaired tooth mineralization and defective metabolism of calcium and phosphate [17]. Hypocalcification, an example of defective low calcification was reported in Indonesian individuals with Down syndrome (DS) [18]. To identify chromosome influence on mineralization, Keinan et al. [19] estimated Ca/P ratios in enamel and dentin of exfoliated and extracted lower second primary molars of children with DS, cerebral palsy (CP) and a control group with no adverse medical history. They revealed that the prenatal levels of enamel formed and the mineralization of enamel of the mesial cusps in DS and CP teeth were significantly lower than that of the control group. Further, growth and mineralization of all cusps were found affected in the teeth of DS. It is therefore, opined that determination of Ca/P ratios in the exfoliated deciduous teeth of developmentally challenged children may aid in finding out the inception and severity of growth abnormalities in utero and their retarding effects on later development of teeth [19].

2.3 Loss of amelogenin gene and mineralization

Amelogenin proteins are essential for the normal development of enamel and are products of ameloblast cells and the primary composition of mineralizing organic matrix of enamel, that becomes mineralized with a hydroxyapatite phase to become the mature enamel [20–22]. The gene loci for human amelogenin, the major protein component of the organic matrix in enamel are on both the X and Y chromosomes [23]. Particularly, the amelogenin genes (AMGX and AMGY) that are identified respectively on the X and Y chromosomes, take part in a prominent role at the time of dental enamel development [24] and exert biologic functions as signaling molecules through cell-surface receptors [25]. When one X-chromosome is absent or malfunctioning in Turner syndrome (TS), expression of the X-chromosome was investigated for mineral incorporation during amelogenesis and indirectly during dentinogenesis. Primary tooth enamel and dentin from girls with TS were analyzed with the use of X-ray microanalysis, microradiography and rule induction analysis and compared with that of healthy girls [26]. High levels of calcium and phosphorus, and low levels of carbon, were found in both TS enamel and dentin; a lower degree of mineralization found in TS enamel is ascribed to low values of carbon. Thus, it is evident that the absence of amelogenin gene (AMGX) expression of the X-chromosome has affected on formation of dental hard tissue.

2.4 Exon4 amelogenins transcription and enamel biomineralization

Amelogenins are proteins formed by alternative splicing of the amelogenin gene and are essential for tooth enamel formation [27, 28]. In a study, Stahl et al. [29] demonstrated the spatiotemporal position of amelogenins, a derivative from transcripts having exon4 (AMG+4) in the enamel matrix and the relative binding of recombinant AMG+4 to hydroxyapatite. Besides, they illustrated that secretion of AMG+4 proteins into the enamel matrix occurred at an early maturation stage and that binding of recombinant AMG+4 to hydroxyapatite was more as compared to binding of recombinant AMG-4. The spatiotemporal site of amelogenins containing exon4 peptide, and their functional variation in hydroxyapatite binding, indicated that the inimitable features of amelogenins having exon4 was responsible for an explicit increase of biomineralization connected to stabilization of early-formed hydroxyapatite at the maturation stage [29].

2.5 Genes and tooth development

Genes above 300 are found in regulating various stages of tooth development [30]. Main genes associated with tooth development include homeobox, MSX, DLX, PAX group and their mutation causes tooth deformity and development disorders [31]. Ogawa et al. [32] and Kapadia et al. [33] **showed that Pax9 controls Msx1 expression and acts with Msx1 at the protein level to activate Msx1 and Bmp4 expression at the time of tooth development.** Expression of KROX-26 gene was identified in the epithelial tissues of the developing tooth during the early bud and cap stages of the growing fetus [34]. **Further,** in human beings, the mutation of MSX, DLX genes [35] and AXIN2 [36] are related to certain syndromes (tooth agenesis and tricho-dento-osseous (TDO) syndrome) and hypodontia or oligodontia. To establish relationships between the syndromes of TDO and the expression patterns of MSX-2, DLX-5, and DLX-7 homeogenes in dentition, Davideau et al. [37] investigated the variation in expression of these three genes and compared their activities in orofacial samples of 7.5–9 week old human embryos. They reported two different patterns of gene expression in different tissues; (1) a stronger gene (MSX-2) expression in the progenitor cells of human orofacial skeletal structures namely bones of mandible and maxilla, Meckel's cartilage, and tooth germs and (2) other two gene expression (DLX-5, DLX-7) only in vestibular lamina and vestibular part of dental epithelium. When the expression patterns of the three genes (MSX-2, DLX-5, and DLX-7) were correlated to the various human tooth types of early development stages, it was discerned that there existed expression of the homeogene in spatially ordered sequences along the vestibular/lingual axis of dental epithelial tissues and different organizing centers involved in the control of human tooth morphogenesis [37].

3. Influences of elements

3.1 Calcium

Insufficient dietary calcium and a reduction in the calcium: phosphorous ratio may promote bone reabsorption, risk of osteoporosis and periodontal disease and increased calcium intake is associated with alleviation of suffering from inflammatory processes, tooth mobility in patients of gingivitis with haemorrhaging [38]. Hence, enough calcium intake is suggested for patients suffering from periodontal disease and to help in the prevention of osteoporosis. Calcium is a key component of the mineralized enamel matrix, but may also have a role in ameloblast cell differentiation. In a study, Chen et al. [39] used human ameloblast lineage cells to determine the effect of calcium on cell function. Primary human ameloblast lineage cells were isolated from human fetal tooth buds and were treated with calcium ranging from 0.05 mM to 1.8 mM. Enhancing calcium levels resulted in notably decreased proliferation of ameloblast cells. The pretreatment of calcium at of 0.1 mM and 0.3 mM concentrations to the cultures caused respectively overexpression of amelogenin, amelotin and type I collagen and formation of a mineralized matrix. Thus, Chen et al. [39], by culturing in vitro human ameloblast lineage cells, showed that the addition of calcium at 0.1 mM and 0.3 mM, induced cell differentiation and upregulation of amelogenin type I collagen and amelotin.

Cementoblasts are tooth root lining cells that are essential for formation of cementum on the root surface and for creating a functional periodontal ligament [40]. Cementoblasts share phenotypical features with osteoblasts. When the increased concentration of extracellular Ca^{2+} is linked to stimulating proliferation and differentiation of osteoblasts, the influence of extracellular Ca^{2+} signaling in cementogenesis has been reported by Kanaya et al. [41]. Using reverse transcription polymerase chain reaction (RT-PCR), they found that enhanced levels of extracellular Ca^{2+} increased fibroblast growth factor (FGF)-2 gene expression.

3.1.1 Calcium sensing receptor gene

Mathias et al. [42] reported that Ca^{2+} may regulate tooth formation and the Ca^{2+}-sensing receptor (CaSR) that is expressed in bone and cartilage has indicated a mechanism by which extracellular Ca^{2+} can regulate cell function. They identified CaSR protein and messenger ribonucleic acide (mRNA) in an immortalized ameloblast-like cell line (PABSo-E) and the expression of CaSR in cultured ameloblasts. In PABSo-E cells, increasing extracellular Ca^{2+} in the medium from 0 (baseline) to 2.5 mM or 5.0 mM resulted in an increase in intracellular Ca^{2+} above baseline to 534 +/− 69 mM and 838 +/− 86 mM, respectively. They revealed that enhancement of Ca^{2+} concentration in the medium could induce the intracellular Ca^{2+} signal transduction pathway and that the CaSR is expressed in developing teeth and may provide a mechanism by which these cells can react to changes in extracellular Ca^{2+} to regulate cell function and eventually, tooth formation. Further, Spurr [43] indicated several sites of expression and functions for the CaSR gene, which includes a role in tooth development and fluid regulation.

3.1.2 Pathway of tricalcium silicate induced gene expression for biomineralization

Calcium-silicate cement is used as a liner and a dentin substitute base under definitive restorative materials [44]. Hence, Du et al. [45] aimed to study tricalcium silicate (C_3S) driven pathway of extracellular signal-regulated kinase 1/2 (ERK1/2) and its role in influencing proliferation and biomineralization occurring in human dental pulp cells (hDPCs) in vitro. They cultured hDPCs in a medium containing C_3S for comparing with controls without C_3S and for measuring biomineralization, cell viability and phosphorylated ERK1/2. The ERK1/2 inhibitor U0126 was used to assess the role of this pathway on stage of the cell cycle and mineralization-dependent gene expressions of hDPCs by using flow cytometry and RT-PCR, respectively. It was observed that C_3S extracts promoted ($P < 0.05$) biomineralization and viability of hDPCs. When hDPCs were cultured in the medium of C_3S extracts, phosphorylated ERK1/2 was noticed within half an hour time. Furthermore, proliferation and the expression of mineralization-dependent genes, including collagen type I, dentin sialophosphoprotein, osteopontin, and osteocalcin were found decreased ($P < 0.05$) due to inhibition of the ERK1/2 pathway by inhibitor U0126 [45]. In conclusion, C_3S stimulated the proliferation and biomineralization of hDPCs in vitro, through the ERK1/2 pathway.

3.2 Roles of calcium of MTA

Mineral trioxide aggregate (MTA), a therapeutic, endodontic repair substance, is associated with activities of tissue calcification even though its mode of action needs further clarification [46]. In order to observe calcium release, calcification activity, calcium-sensing receptor (CaSR) gene expression and bone morphogenetic protein-2 (BMP-2), and BMP-2 receptor protein and gene expression, two populations of human periodontal ligament cells (HPLCs) that were donated by two patients, were cultured in the presence or absence of MTA discs and/or $CaCl_2$ [47]. It was found out that within 2 weeks MTA released a considerable concentration of calcium (4 mmol/L) into culture media. HPLCs innately exhibited gene expression encoding for the receptors of CaSR and BMP-2. Supplementation of exogenous

$CaCl_2$ in the media effected expression of CaSR gene, calcification and BMP-2 synthesis during the whole HPLC cultures, while supplementation of magnesium chloride yielded no impact on mineralization and gene expression. Maeda et al. [47] concluded that HPLCs cocultured directly with MTA up-regulated BMP2 expression and calcification.

3.3 Calcium and phosphorus

Several culture systems with human dental pulp cells are employed to find out the mechanisms involved in dentin formation through promotion of differentiation of dental pulp (DP) cells into odontoblasts [48, 49]. When explants from human teeth were cultured in Eagle's basal medium supplemented with 10% or 15% fetal calf serum, with or without beta-glycerophosphate (beta GP), Couble et al. [48] reported that addition of beta GP to the culture medium induced odontoblast features in the cultured pulp cells. Further, they showed through splendid structural evaluation of the cultured pulp cell that the presence of typical intracellular organelles was manifested in the body of odontoblast and afterward there appeared an area of mineralization in type I collagen rich matrix. The presence of calcium and phosphorus was evident from X-ray microanalysis while the apatite crystal structure of the mineral was confirmed through electron diffraction pattern. Finally, two patterns of expression were identified, viz., elevated expression of alpha 1(1) collagen mRNAs in all polarized cells and dentin sialoprotein gene expression in mineralizing areas including their association with calcium and phosphorus [48].

3.4 Calcium, magnesium and enamel formation genes

A genetic component in caries susceptibility is related to variation in enamel formation genes [50]. The trends of tooth demineralization and remineralization in a group of subjects are related to chosen five genes (ENAM (enamelin), MMP20 (matrix metalloproteinase 20), TUFT (tuftelin), TFIP (tuftelin-interacting protein), and AMBN (amelobalstin)). In a study, Halusic et al. [51] exposed primary baseline teeth (20 h) to an artificial caries solution as well as remineralizing solution to measure Ca and Mg concentrations in the biopsies of three categories of baseline, carious, and fluoridated teeth and to compare these tooth categories with allele and genotype frequencies for calcium and magnesium levels. Halusic et al. [51] pointed out that calcium content was higher than magnesium levels in each sample and there existed associations of genetic variation of only two genes, ENAM and AMBN with mineral concentrations. As a result, it is substantiated that there exits obvious association among influencing roles of enamel formation genes, tooth levels of calcium and magnesium and the caries development.

3.5 Selenium from dental material for stronger teeth

Selenium, an essential trace element is a constituent of antioxidant enzymes [52] and can replace sulphur in bonds of collagen resulting in stronger Se-collagen bond than a sulphur bond. Since collagen is the most important component of the organic matrix of the tooth and Se-collagen bond is stronger, the beneficial role of selenium is evident from stronger teeth of children and adults [53]. Dental filling materials are one of selenium sources of body intake and its additional benefits were tested in the experimental tooth samples of 60 subjects who were treated with endodontic dressing in the following four groups: selenium (Se), calcium hydroxide, calcium hyrdoxide + selenium and controls without Se (n = 15) [54]. With use of RT-PCR, expression of the prokaryotic 16S ribosomal RNA and microbial growth were evaluated before cleaning and shaping procedures and after 15 days of treatment of the groups with or without filling materials. The finding of the evaluation indicated that selenium use from the source of tooth material filling was significantly effective in reducing the microbial growth by decreasing the IFN-γ mRNA expression for healthy strong teeth [54].

3.6 Strontium

Strontium is recognized as a most recent version of anti-osteoporotic agent that causes immediately anti-catabolic and anabolic effects on bone cells [55]. Römer et al. [56] employed strontium in vitro to explore its application to promote bone marker transcription and hydroxyapatite formation on isolated Runx2 (Runt-related transcription factor 2) osteoblasts samples of subjects with a disease of cleidocranial dysplasia. This ailment is caused owing to insufficient gene dosage and heterozygous mutations of Runx2 which is an essential transcription factor 2 for maturing of osteoblast and transcription of osteogenic genes. This genetic deficiency is attributed to supernumerary teeth, aplasia or hypoplasia of clavicles, symptoms of hypophosphatasia (HPP) and patent fontanelles. In an investigation, Römer et al. [56] aimed to examine strontium influence on the formation of hydroxyapatite, the cell proliferation of strontium-treated Runx2 osteoblasts and gene expression of bone marker proteins. The results of their study manifested improved hydroxyapatite formation in the extracellular matrix and gene expression of bone marker proteins in strontium-treated Runx2 osteoblasts. A water soluble tetrazolium salts-1 cell proliferation assay with strontium-treated Runx2 osteoblasts indicated that cell proliferation and growth were promoted by strontium. As a consequence of strontium inducing effects, enhanced mineralization of the extracellular matrix was recognized in the strontium-treated Runx2(+/−)-osteoblasts.

When strontium forms a significant component of dental restorative materials and is widely used in toothpastes, Huang et al. [57] mentioned that low dose Sr (between 0.1 and 2.5 mM) induced proliferation and alkaline phosphatase (ALP) activity, collagen formation and mineralization of human dental pulp stem cells (hDPSC) in vitro. With the use of quantitative reverse transcription polymerase chain reaction (qRT-PCR), Western blotting and immunocytochemistry techniques in hDPSCs, strontium was found regulating gene expression and the protein secretion of the odontogenic markers (dentine sialophosphoprotein), dentine matrix protein 1, calcium sensing receptor, the downstream pathway of MAPK and ERK signaling pathway. Strontium specifically in the bioavailable form from bioglass (BG) appeared regulating metabolic and alkaline phosphate activities in hDPSCs. Henceforth, it is viewed that the element, strontium at definite concentrations considerably gives rise to odontogenic differentiation, proliferation and mineralization of hDPSCs in vitro through calcium-sensing receptor resembling to the pathway of osteoblast differentiation [57]. It is suggested based on these findings that Sr treatment of hDPSCs could be a promising therapeutic agent in dental applications and that Sr from a substituted BG could be used more effectively in biomaterials designed for dental applications.

3.7 Strontium phosphate

In another study, Su et al. [58] found out that strontium phosphate had an impact on the osteogenic differentiation of SHEDs (stem cells from human exfoliated deciduous teeth); especially, the action of the phosphate compound was linked to improved osteogenic differentiation of SHEDs along with elevated expression of the osteoblast-related genes. Two modes of activities were reported on chitosan scaffolds containing strontium, namely (1) reduced proliferation of SHEDs and (2) notably increased activities of type-I collagen expression, alkaline phosphatase role, and calcium deposition. Therefore, it is proposed that strontium has an important function in tooth remodeling because it can simulate tooth formation and decrease resorption.

3.8 Strontium ranelate

Tian et al. [59] in research, produced strontium ranelate-loaded chitosan film on titanium surfaces with five values of strontium ranelate (SR) (0, 2, 20, 40, and 80 mmol/L of the strontium ion [Sr^{2+}]) to find Sr^{2+} effects of bone healing. The low levels of 2 mmol/L or 20 mmol/L of SR loaded onto the chitosan film caused improved cell responses of primary oestoblasts (POBs) with obvious proliferation, alkaline phosphatase (ALP) activity, and expression of bone morphogenetic protein 2 (BMP-2), runt-related transcription factor 2 (Runx2), ALP, and osteocalcin, whereas SR at great values of 40 mmol/L or 80 mmol/L suppressed the growth of POBs. The conclusive finding is that the SR-imbibed chitosan film on a titanium exterior surface supports proliferation and differentiation of osteoblasts in a concentration-dependent way and the subsequent recommendation is that strontium and titanium have definite utilities as safe implant materials of dental treatment [59].

Osteoporosis that is caused due to intensified bone loss, is associated with periodontitis and the two have the general causal factors of bone resorption [60]. One of the strategies commonly practiced to deal with the illness of periodontitis is that when SR is used, strontium ions released from SR, involves in an explicit influence on arresting activation of osteoclast and inducing differentiation of osteoblast. Jia et al. [61] studied the processes of periodontal regeneration promoted by strontium and elucidated that the epigenetic mechanism of splicing factor, heterogeneous nuclear ribonucleoprotein L (hnRNPL) promoted osteogenesis processing of periodontal ligament stem cells (PDLSCs) that were activated by strontium chloride. When SET domain containing 2 is an enzyme that in humans is encoded by the SETD2 gene and hnRNPL has osteogenesis promotion, there are chances of utilizing strontium, hnRNPL and SET domain containing 2 for curing periodontitis patients concurrently ailing from osteoporosis [61].

3.9 Iron role in cytodifferentiation of human periodontal ligament cells

The periodontal ligament (PDL) is essential in maintaining homeostasis of tooth and periodontal tissue [62] and iron overload or deficiency can have adverse impacts on alveolar bone density. In a study, the requirement of iron levels for the cytodifferentiation of PDL cells was reported by Hou et al. [63]. After supplementing in a culture medium of human PDL cells with 10–50 μm ammonium ferric citrate or 5 μm deferoxamine (an iron chelator) during differentiation, the status of intracellular iron was measured by determining the level of expression of ferritin RNA and protein; in addition, the differentiation and function of PDL cells were assessed by estimating osteoblast differentiation gene markers and the capability of formation of mineralized nodules in the culture. The results of the study indicated that the accumulation of iron caused increased regulation of light and heavy chain ferritin protein. Concomitantly, inhibition of osteoblast differentiation gene markers and mineralized nodule formation appeared in the culture medium. Deficiency of iron occurred during PDL cell differentiation led to decreased three activities namely (1) downregulation of both the light and heavy chain ferritin proteins, (2) diminished alkaline phosphatase activity and (3) poor mineralized nodule formation. Thus, it is concluded that iron is critical for the normal cell differentiation of human PDL cells [63].

3.10 Potassium hydrogen phosphate in mineralization

Stem cells from dental apical papilla (SCAPs) can be induced to differentiate along both osteoblast and odontoblast lineages [64] and effect of KH2PO4 was studied on differentiation efficiency in SCAPs by Wang et al. [65]. Stem cells that were isolated from apical papillae of immature third molars were exposed to two kinds of mineralization-inducing media, MM1 and MM2, with two different concentrations of KH_2PO_4. The levels of proliferation and osteo/odontogenic differentiation of SCAPs were correlated between MM1 and MM2 treatments. Investigation with cell counting and flow cytometry revealed that the proliferative potential of SCAPs was greater in MM2 containing 1.8 mM additional KH_2PO_4 than in MM1. Similarly, the SCAPs were much better in MM2 medium than in MM1 for various higher activities such as osteo/odontogenesis, alkaline phosphatase activity, calcium deposition and expression of osteo/odontoblast-specific genes/proteins (e.g., runt-related transcription factor 2, and osteocalcin). When KH_2PO_4 1.8 mM was added into the media, there were positive effects of notably increased cell proliferation, better differentiation capacity of SCAPs along osteo/odontogenic cell lineages and enhanced mineralization, in comparison to control media lacking additional KH_2PO_4 [65].

3.11 Effect of phosphate

Mutations in the gene ALPL in hypophosphatasia (HPP) decreased activities of tissue nonspecific alkaline phosphatase and the consequent rise in pyrophosphate (PP(i)) caused bone and tooth mineralization malfunction by affecting calcium-phosphate (P(i)) precipitation [66]. To find out mechanisms involved in HPP-associated pulp/dentin phenotypes, Rodrigues et al. [67] cultured primary pulp cells from hypophosphatasia (HPP) subjects to assay alkaline phosphatase (ALP) activity, mineralization, and gene expression for comparison with cells from healthy controls. Exogenous P(i) was provided to the correct P(i)/PP(i) ratio in cell culture. The results of the culture studies demonstrated that HPP cells showed remarkably lower ALP activity (by 50%) and mineral nodule formation (by 60%) than the activities of controls. The affected expression of PP(i) regulatory genes was found in the HPP pulp cells, including a decrease in the progressive ankylosis gene (ANKH) and high ectonucleotide pyrophosphatase/phosphodiesterase 1 (ENPP1). P(i) supplementation in the culture restored a remedial activity for the mineralization and moderately rescued a few gene expressions, even though the cells had already changed messenger RNA contents for PP(i)-connected genes. Rodrigues et al. [67] opined that low mineralization and disrupted odontoblast profile caused in pulp cells under HPP conditions, were the first steps of the molecular mechanisms for dentin phenotypes observed in HPP.

3.12 Aluminum oxide particles

Periodontal ligament stem cells (PDLSCs) are capable of regenerating the periodontal tissues including alveolar bone tissue [68]. Further, PDLSCs being considered as the stem cells are associated with the osseointegration of titanium implants, immediately after an implant is fixed in the fresh gap of the extracted socket. Therefore, Heo et al. [69] cultured PDLSCs on three sorts of titanium surface textures ((1) smooth machined, (2) blasted with 75 and 125 μm Al_2O_3 particles, and (3) anodized) to check their proliferation and gene expressions of osteocalcin, osteopontin, type I collagen, and GAPDH. From these experiments, Heo et al. [69] proposed three deliberations namely, (1) elevated proliferation of PDLSCs on the rough surface blasted with 75 μm Al_2O_3 particles, (2) increased osteocalcin expression on the Al_2O_3 particle treated-surface regardless of its particle size and generally lowered type I collagen expression with time in 6 days culture. In conclusion, titanium surface coating has inducing effects of Al_2O_3 due to greater proliferation of PDLSCs in the culture and higher expression of osteocalcin.

3.13 Phosphate of Mg, Sr and Zn and chloride of Mg

Divalent Mg, Sr and Zn contribute significantly to bone remodeling through osteoinductivity because of their roles in inducing bone formation and reducing bone resorption [70, 71]. So, Huang et al. [72] experimented to examine the impacts of a few divalent metal phosphates on osteogenic differentiation from human exfoliated deciduous teeth by steadily releasing the divalent metal ions from the scaffold into the culture medium and repetitively activating osteoblastic differentiation. They reported that osteoblastic differentiation was conspicuously higher in the SHEDs cultured within chitosan scaffolds containing the phosphates of divalent metals than in the cells cultured without the phosphates of metals. The observed metal influence was attributed to elevated action of alkaline phosphatase and also the bone-related gene expression of collagen type I, Runx2, osteopontin, osteocalcin, VEGF, and Ang-1, which were evident from the technique of RT-PCR and immunocytochemistry staining of bone-related protein [72]. A noteworthy enrichment of deposited minerals, especially the phosphates of Mg and Zn, which were discerned on the scaffolds after 21 days of culture, was apparent from a calcium-content assay. Similarly, $MgCl_2$ at 10 mM concentration increased odontogenic differentiation in human dental pulp stem cells by promoting ERK/BMP2/Smads signaling through enrichment of intracellular magnesium [73]. It is, therefore, concluded and recommended that except barium phosphate, other metal (Sr, Mg and Zn) phosphates and $MgCl_2$ which are found effectively promoting SHED cell differentiation and osteoblastic cell maturation, have significant efficacy and immense utility in tissue engineering and bone repair.

3.14 Ca^{2+}, Gd^{3+}, Sr^{2+}, or Al^{3+}

Kanaya et al. [41] showed that treatment with trivalent/divalent inorganic ions, Ca^{2+}, Gd^{3+}, Sr^{2+} and Al^{3+} except Mg^{2+} in cementoblasts (tooth root lining cells) resulted in a dose-dependent elevation of fibroblast growth factor (FGF-2) mRNA levels in a cAMP-dependent fashion. Because of this finding, it is presumed that a mechanism of extracellular Ca^{2+}-sensing exists in the cementoblasts and its regulation results in FGF-2 activation in a cAMP/PKA dependent manner. The knowledge of the pathway leading to primary genes' expression for modulating the regeneration of oral tissues will guide in making use of these inorganic elements and designing regenerative therapies in dentistry. In support, the regenerative capacity of dental pulp stem cells was found higher due to higher osteocalcin and the Runx2 gene expression caused by the scaffolds containing Sr_2 and Ce_3 [74].

3.15 Manganese effects on *Streptococcus mutans* virulence gene expression

Comparison of trace metals in drinking water with that of tooth enamel has led to prediction of a caries-influencing role of manganese (Mn) [75]. Manganese, an essential element, is required for the expression of mutant *Streptococci sobrinus*'s virulence factors, glucan-binding lectin (GBL) whose functional analogue is a glucan-binding protein (Gbps/GbpC) that is found contributing to biofilm architecture and virulence. Therefore, Arirachakaran et al. [76] explored the effects of Mn on the transcription of genes encoding *Streptococcus mutans* (*S. mutans*) Gbps, including GbpC, along with other critical *S. mutans* virulence genes for understanding Mn role in mutant induced tooth caries. With the use of northern and western blots and RT-PCR techniques, they aimed to find the differences of Mn impacts on the selected Gbp genes under conditions of planktonic and biofilm cultures of *S. mutans* in media with 50 μM Mn and without Mn. Their findings showed different forms of Mn effects namely, (1) increased expression of GbpC and gtfB, (2) decreased expression of wapA, in both planktonic and biofilm cultures, (3) decreased expression of GbpA and GbpD only in biofilms and (4) increased expression of gtfC only in planktonic cultures [76]. Thus, it is delineated that Mn availability affects the expression of multiple *S. mutans* genes involved in adhesion and biofilm formation.

3.16 Boron and molecular mechanism of gene expression

Boron is an essential micronutrient participating in metabolism and a few boron derivatives are found promoting the growth of bone and teeth in vivo [77]. So, Taşlı et al. [78] studied molecular mechanism of bone formation, while evaluating cell differentiation and toxicity of sodium pentaborate pentahydrate (NaB) at various concentrations. Further, they assessed odontogenic, osteogenic differentiation and biomineralization of human tooth germ stem cells (hTGSCs) by measuring the levels of mRNA expression, odontogenic and osteogenic protein expression, alkaline phosphatase (ALP) activity, mineralization, and calcium deposits. In comparison to control, the hTGSCs exposed to NaB showed the uppermost ALP activity and expression of osteo- and odontogenic-related genes and proteins. Since NaB has the functional role of promoting in vitro odontogenic and osteogenic differentiation, it is viewed as a promising compound for the development of new scaffold systems in both bone and tooth tissue engineering [78].

3.17 Lead

Lead (Pb^{2+}) exposure continues to be a significant public health problem and teeth have been recognized as a useful long-term record of lead (Pb^{2+}) uptake [79, 80]. Thaweboon et al. [81] cultured dental pulp cells (DP cells) from the teeth of young patients (aged 17–24 years) and treated them with lead glutamate to examine in vitro effects of lead on DP cells. The results of their study denoted that in serum-free conditions lead at all three concentrations (4.5×10^{-5} M, 4.5×10^{-6} M, and 4.5×10^{-7} M) caused radically enhanced proliferation of DP cells and only one lead concentration of 4.5×10^{-5} M and in 2% fetal bovine serum caused increasing cell proliferation. But the significantly decreased levels of protein, procollagen type I, and osteocalcin secretion observed are indicative of the affected state of DP cells and toxic effects of lead.

In another in vitro study, stem cells obtained from primary and secondary teeth, and periodontal ligament were exposed to five concentrations of lead nitrate (160, 80, 40, 20, and 10 μM) for 24 hours to find out its adverse impacts on the proliferation, differentiation, and gene expression in these cell lines [82]. The findings of the study revealed damaging lead effects viz., (1) altered morphology and adhesion of the cells in a concentration-dependent fashion, (2) a severe downregulation of osteogenesis and ectoderm and endoderm markers, demonstrating an irregular and untimely differentiation trail and (3) a regular expression of key markers associated with stemness (Oct 4, Rex 1) and DNA repair enzyme markers. Abdullah et al. [82] conclusively corroborated the harmful lead effects of modified differentiation and expression of the stem cells.

3.18 Titanium

Titanium is also another element finding its way from dental alloy into the oral cavity to cause various effects. Peri-implant granulation tissue fibroblasts (PIGFs) were exposed to TiO_2 particles, *Porphyromonas gingivalis* and a mixture of TiO_2 particles and *P. gingivalis* to determine gene expression and protein production of pro-inflammatory mediators by PIGFs with the use of the techniques of PCR and enzyme-linked immunoassay (ELISA) [83]. It was observed that at high concentration TiO_2 was toxic to PIGFs and at sub-toxic level, it promoted high gene expression of tumour necrosis factor A (TNF-A) and enhanced protein production of TNF-α, interleukin (IL)-6 and IL-8. Both TiO_2 particles and *P. gingivalis* caused higher effects than *P. gingivalis* alone. In another investigation, Wang et al. [84] observed that after treatment with submicron particles of titanium, human mesenchymal stem cells showed reduced levels of several activities namely, bone sialoprotein (BSP) gene expression, collagen type I and BSP production, cellular proliferation and viability and matrix mineralization. Further, Salvi et al. [85] revealed that incorporation of titanium dental implants into hard and soft tissue resulted in a multifarious biological activities viz., osseointegration linked to inflammation and a raise of gene expression for osteogenesis, angiogenesis and neurogenesis of wound healing.

Global DNA methylation was determined in 21 subjects with peri-implantitis and 24 subjects with healthy implants with use of immunohistochemical measurement of 5-methylcytosine (5mC) in peri-implant crevicular fluid samples and related to titanium levels analysed with inductively coupled plasma mass spectrometry (ICP-MS) in submucosal plaque samples [86]. The levels of 5mC were notably greater in peri-implantitis samples than the healthy implant samples ($P = 0.002$). Therefore, it is opined that there is a relationship between peri-implantitis and epigenetic alterations in the peri-implant tissues and that methylation may be affected by titanium dissolution products. In conclusion, it viewed that because of corrosion and deposition from implants, titanium toxicity may pose at gene level several tooth weakening effects namely, inflammation, allergy, bone loss, failure of osseointegration and dental implants [87].

3.19 Nickel

Nickel becomes a source from alloys of dental application and causes intraoral metal contact allergy [88, 89], inflammatory response [90, 91] and cytotoxicity [92] that are associated with the expression of different genes described as follows. X-ray fluorescence microscopy and spectrometry for measurement of metal level released from the alloy, histochemical analysis, RT-PCR and western blotting for the expression level of HLA-DR were employed to compare between gingival tissues collected from the subjects with allergy and affected by alloy restoration and normal gingival tissue samples [88]. The allergic groups showed significantly higher levels of protein and gene expression of human leukocyte antigen DR (HLA-DR) than ($P < 0.01$) control group without any metal exposure [88]. In allergic patients metals of alloys are responsible for inducing HLA-DR which is one of the major histocompatibility complex class II antigens and associated with antigen presentation to CD_4^+ T lymphocytes [93].

In a study reported by Li et al. [91], impacts of nickel(II) on the expression of inflammatory cytokine, receptor genes and nuclear factor-kappa B (NFκB)-related genes were determined by using qRT-PCR and PCR-based arrays in the human THP1 monocytic cell line pre-exposed to Ni(II) for 72 h. Both downregulation of 10 inflammatory genes and up-regulation of IL8 and seven NFκB-related genes' expression were found induced by Ni(II) only in the pre-exposed group. Wylie et al. [90] treated H400 oral keratinocytes with two Ni-based dental alloys (Matchmate and Dsign10) and $NiCl_2$ (1–40 μg/mL Ni^{2+}) and found that exposure to increasing concentrations of $NiCl_2$ decreased cell growth and morphology and increased all cytokine transcripts at 1 day. On day 6, IL-1beta and IL-8 transcripts were negatively affected, whereas granulocyte-macrophage colony-stimulating factor (GM-CSF) and IL-11 enhanced with Ni^{2+} dose. Further, Messer and Lucas [92] indicated that Ni ions released from alloys affected several cellular functions and their cytotoxic effects relied on the factors namely ion chemistry, ion valence, and dose-time dependence. In conclusion, it is viewed that there exist the main concerns about biocompatibility of harmful nickel ions released from the alloys into dental and surrounding tissues [92].

3.20 Mineralization and genes

The human *TUFT1* gene is expressed at the time of development and mineralization of enamel through coding for tuftelin, a glycoprotein identified in enamel [94, 95]. Halusic et al. [51] reported that among the selected genes, ENAM, MMP20, TUFT, TFIP, and AMBN, only two genes EAM and AMBN were found associated with calcium mineralization, whereas Jeremias et al. [96] reported a significant association of 3 genes (*TFIP11*, *ENAM*, and *AMELX*) with molar-incisor hypomineralization.

Pang et al. [50] have used a *Streptococcus mutans* biofilm model to verify if variants in genes are connected with mineral loss in dental enamel. In the samples of saliva and enamels from 213 individuals, they carried out DNA extraction and analyses of 16 single nucleotide polymorphisms in the saliva and also analyses of physical and chemical properties, mineral loss and the lesion depth of the demineralized enamel samples under cariogenic challenge for comparison between different genotypes at each single nucleotide polymorphism. Their findings pointed out the genes associated with minerals both at higher levels [Mn in GG genotype of AMBN (rs7694409), Ca in GT genotype of MMP20 (rs1612069), Ca/P ratio in GG genotype of AMBN (rs13115627)] and also at lower levels [Mn in CT genotype of TFIP11 (rs2097470) and P in GG genotype of AMBN (rs13115627), AG genotype of ENAM (rs12640848) and AA genotype of MMP20 (rs2292730)]. Subsequently, the lower mineral levels were connected with the mineral loss, depth loss and the genes (TFIP11, TUFT1, MMP20, and ENAM). They suggested that genetic variations in the genes of TFIP11, TUFT1, MMP20, and ENAM influenced enamel demineralization in a *Streptococcus mutans* biofilm model and the possibilities of weakening the tooth structure due to demineralizing action of certain genes [50].

4. Summary and conclusions

Elements are found influencing mineralization, cell differentiation and development of teeth. Differences in the effects of elements are associated with ionic and compound forms and dose. Their influence is through gene expression. **Table 1** shown the various elements' influence on gene expression associated with the mineralization, cell differentiation and tooth development. Prominently four kinds of gene expressions were reported, namely up regulation by B, Ca, Sr, Fe, K, P, $MgCl_2$, Divalent ions (Mg, Zn, etc.), down-regulation by tricalcium silicate and lead, no expression by barium phosphate and adverse gene expression by lead nitrate. Broadly the effects could be positive, neutral and negative correspondingly related to their types as essential, non-essential and harmful elements which are to be considered

SN	Element/compound	Stem cells used	Method used	Gene identified	Nature of gene expression & [reference]
1	Ca^{2+}, Gd^{3+}, Sr^{2+}, Al^{3+}	Cementoblast	RT-PCR	Fibroblast growth factor (FGF)-2 gene	Increase in FGF-2 expression [41]
2	Ca from MTA	Human periodontal ligament cells	In vitro & gene expression techniques	Calcium-sensing receptor (CaSR) gene	Increase in gene expression [47]
3	Ca	Human ameloblast lineage cells	Techniques of PCR, Immunoassay, phase contrast microscope	AMELX, COL1A1, AMTN	Upregulated expression of amelogenin, type I collagen & amelotin [39]
4	Se	Intracanal dental cells	RT-PCR	IFN-γ mRNA expression	Down regulated IFN-γ expression for anti-inflammation [54]
5	Sr	Runx2(+/−) osteoblasts	RNA isolation, RT-PCR, fluorescence staining & quantification, cell growth analysis & WST-1 cell proliferation test	Runx2	Improved mineralisation of the extracellular matrix [56]
6	Sr	Human dental pulp stem cells	qRT-PCR, western blotting and immune-cytochemistry techniques	(DSPP) and dentine matrix protein 1 (DMP-1) genes	Proliferation, odontogenic differentiation and mineralisation of hDPSCs [57]
7	Strontium phosphate	Stem cells from human exfoliated deciduous teeth	Osteogenic differentiation, RT-PCR, alkaline phosphatase assay, calcium quantification, perfusion dynamic culture	Osteoblast-related gene	Up-regulated expression for enhanced cellular differentiation [58]
8	Strontium ranelate	Primary oestoblasts	X-ray diffraction, scanning electron microscopy, Fourier transform infrared spectroscopy	Osteoblastic gene	Promotes osteoblast proliferation and differentiation [59]
9	Strontium ranelate	Periodontal ligament stem cells	Immune-histochemistry, western blotting, RNA extraction, RT-qPCR	Heterogeneous nuclear ribonucleo-protein L-gene	Preventing osteoclast & promoting osteoblast differentiation [61]
10	Iron	Human periodontal ligament cells	Techniques of measurements of ferritin RNA and protein, gene expression	Osteoblast differentiation gene	Fe is critical for normal differentiation of human PDL cells [63]
11	Potassium hydrogen phosphate	Stem cells from the dental apical papilla	Flow cytometry, alkaline phosphatase assay, alizarin red staining, TR-PCR, western blot, immune-cytochemistry	Osteo/odontoblast-specific genes	Upregulated gene expression for enhanced cell growth & improved differentiation [65]
12	P	Primary pulp cells from hypophosphatasia (HPP) subjects	qRT-PCR, von Kossa assay, alizarin red S staining, ALP activity assay	Odontoblast marker genes	P addition enhanced mineralization & rescued some of gene expression [67]

SN	Element/compound	Stem cells used	Method used	Gene identified	Nature of gene expression & [reference]
13	Divalent Mg, Sr, Zn & P	Stem cells from human exfoliated deciduous teeth	RT-PCR, immune-cytochemistry, ALP activity assay	Gene of collagen type-I, Runx2, osteopontin, osteocalcin, VEGF, and Ang-1	High activity of alkaline phosphatase, & high osteoblastic cell maturation & differentiation [72]
14	Boron	Human tooth germ stem cells	RT-PCR, immune-cytochemistry, ALP activity assay	Osteo- and odontogenic related genes	Increased alkaline phosphatase) activity, osteo- & odontogenic differentiation & biomineralization [78]
15	Aluminum oxide particles	Periodontal ligament adult stem cells	RT-PCR, immune-cytochemistry, enzyme activity assay	Genes of osteocalcin, osteopontin, type I collagen & GAPDH	Increased osteocalcin & decreased type I collagen expression [69]
16	$MgCl_2$	Human periodontal ligament cells	RT-PCR	ERK/BMP2/Snads signaling genes	Increased odontogenic differentiation [73]
17	Mg^{2+}	Shed human exfoliated deciduous teeth	RT-PCR, western blot	Genes of collagen type 1, Runx2, osteopontin, osteocalcin, VEGF, and Ang-1,	Elevated gene expression and mineral deposit [72]
18	Barium phosphate	Stem cells from human exfoliated deciduous teeth	RT-PCR, western blot	Genes of collagen type 1, Runx2, osteopontin, osteocalcin, VEGF, and Ang-1,	No effect [73]
19	Tricalcium silicate	Human dental pulp cells	RT-PCR, ALP activity analysis, alizarin red S staining	Mineralization-dependent genes	Decrease of gene expression [45]
20	Lead	Human dental pulp fibroblasts cells of patients	RT-PCR, ALP activity analysis, western blot	Genes of procollagen type I, and osteocalcin	Decreased protein, procollagen type I, and osteocalcin productions [81]
21	Lead nitrate	Stem cells of deciduous & permanent teeth, periodontal ligament & bone marrow	RT-PCR, MTT & LDH assay, immune-phenotyping assay	Genes of Oct 4, Rex 1 and DNA repair enzyme	Alteration in the differentiation and gene expression in the cells [82]
22	Titanium	Peri-implant granulation tissue fibroblasts	PCR & ELISA	TNF-α, IL-6 & IL-8	High gene expression for causing peri-implantitis [83]
23	Nickel	Human THP1 monocytic cells	qRT-PCR	10 inflammatory genes, IL-8 & 7 NFκB-related genes	Up regulation of IL-8 & 7 NFκB-related genes for inflammation [91]

Table 1.
Effects of elements on the genes expression, differentiation and mineralization in the different dental stem cells.

for their multiple sources from diet, environment and dental materials and implants. Besides other properties and utilities, essential elements (Ca, Sr, Se, Cr, Fe, K, P etc.) are included and harmful elements (Pb) are excluded from oral intake and in the composition of dental products formulated and fabricated for multiple requirements in dentistry, whereas Ni and Ti use is continued since their effects of allergy and inflammation are very rare and possibilities of their substitutes are explored.

Acknowledgements

The author thanks the Principal, Regional Institute of Education, Mysore and the Director, National Council of Educational Research and Training, New Delhi, India for their moral support and encouragement.

Author details

Sukumar Athimoolam
Department of Education in Science and Mathematics, Regional Institute of Education, National Council of Educational Research and Training, Mysore, Karnataka, India

*Address all correspondence to: sukumarindia@rediffmail.com

References

[1] Goldberg M, Kulkarni AB, Young M, Boskey A. Dentin: Structure, composition and mineralization: The role of dentin ECM in dentin formation and mineralization. Frontiers in Bioscience. 2011;**3**:711-735

[2] Lin CP, Douglas WH, Erlandsen SL. Scanning electron microscopy of type I collagen at the dentin-enamel junction of human teeth. The Journal of Histochemistry and Cytochemistry. 1993;**41**(3):381-388

[3] Gelse K, Pöschl E, Aigner T. Collagens—structure, function, and biosynthesis. Advanced Drug Delivery Reviews. 2003;**55**(12):1531-1546

[4] Hart S, Hart T. Disorders of human dentin. Cells, Tissues, Organs. 2007;**186**(1):70-77. DOI: 10.1159/000102682

[5] Lacruz RS, Habelitz S, Wright JT, Paine ML. Dental enamel formation and implications for oral health and disease. Physiological Reviews. 2017;**97**(3):939-993. DOI: 10.1152/physrev.00030.2016

[6] Neel A, Aljabo A, Strange A, Ibrahim S, Coathup M, Young AM, et al. Demineralization–remineralization dynamics in teeth and bone. International Journal of Nanomedicine. 2016;**11**:4743-4763

[7] Raj A, Oudenaarden AV. Stochastic gene expression and its consequences. Cell. 2008;**135**(2):216-226. DOI: 10.1016/j.cell.2008.09.050

[8] Rai PK, Lee SS, Zhang M, Tsang YF, Kim KH. Heavy metals in food crops: Health risks, fate, mechanisms, and management. Environment International. 2019;**125**:365-385. DOI: org/10.1016/j.envint.2019.01.067

[9] Maria Cristina LGS, Sergio Roberto PL. The genetics of amelogenesis imperfecta. A review of the literature. Journal of Applied Oral Science. 2005;**13**(3):212-217

[10] Romito A, Cobellis G. Pluripotent stem cells: Current understanding and future directions. Stem Cells International. 2016;**2016**:9451492. DOI:10.1155/2016/9451492

[11] Ullah I, Subbarao RB, Rho GJ. Human mesenchymal stem cells—current trends and future prospective. Bioscience Reports. 2015;**35**(2):e00191. DOI: 10.1042/BSR20150025

[12] Potdar PD, Jethmalani YD. Human dental pulp stem cells: Applications in future regenerative medicine. World Journal Stem Cells. 2015;**7**(5):839-851. DOI: 10.4252/wjsc.v7.i5.839

[13] Yu L, Wei M. Biomineralization of collagen-based materials for hard tissue repair. International Journal of Molecular Sciences. 2021;**22**(2):944. DOI: 10.3390/ijms22020944

[14] Caruso S, Bernardi S, Pasini M, Giuca MR, Docimo R, Continenza MA, et al. The process of mineralisation in the development of human tooth. European Journal of Paediatric Dentistry. 2016;**17**(4):322-326

[15] Goldberg M, Septier D, Lécolle S, Chardin H, Quintana MA, Acevedo AC, et al. Dental mineralization. The International Journal of Developmental Biology. 1995;**39**(1):93-110

[16] Alvesalo L. Sex chromosomes and human growth. A dental approach. Human Genetics. 1997;**101**(1):1-5. DOI: 10.1007/s004390050575

[17] Vital SO, Gaucher C, Bardet C, Rowe PS, George A, Linglart A, et al. Tooth dentin defects reflect genetic disorders affecting bone mineralization. Bone. 2012;**50**(4):989-997. DOI: 10.1016/j.bone.2012.01.010

[18] L Anggraini, MF Rizal, IS Indiart. Prevalence of dental anomalies in indonesian individuals with Down syndrome. Pesquisa Brasileira em Odontopediatria e Clínica Integrada 2019;**19**:e5332. DOI: http://doi.org/10.4034/PBOCI.2019.191.147

[19] Keinan D, Smith P, Zilberman U. Microstructure and chemical composition of primary teeth in children with Down syndrome and cerebral palsy. Archives of Oral Biology. 2006;**51**(10):836-843

[20] Lau EC, Slavkin HC, Snead ML. Analysis of human enamel genes: Insights into genetic disorders of enamel. The Cleft Palate Journal. 1990;**27**(2):121-130

[21] Collier PM, Sauk JJ, Rosenbloom SJ, Yuan ZA, Gibson CW. An amelogenin gene defect associated with human X-linked amelogenesis imperfect. Archives of Oral Biology. 1997;**42**(3):235-242. DOI: 10.1016/s0003-9969(96)00099-4

[22] Frasheri I, Ern C, Diegritz C, Hickel R, Hristov M, Folwaczny M. Full-length amelogenin influences the differentiation of human dental pulp stem cells. Stem Cell Research & Therapy. 2016;7:10. DOI: 10.1186/s13287-015-0269-9

[23] Alvesalo L. Human sex chromosomes in oral and craniofacial growth. Archives of Oral Biology. 2009;**54**(Supplement 1):S18-S24. DOI: 10.1016/j.archoralbio.2008.06.004

[24] Salido EC, Yen PH, Koprivnikar K, Yu LC, Shapiro LJ. The human enamel protein gene amelogenin is expressed from both the X and the Y chromosomes. American Journal of Human Genetics. 1992;**50**(2):303-316

[25] Tanimoto K, Kunimatsu R, Tanne Y, Huang YC, Michida M, Yoshimi Y, et al. Differential effects of amelogenin on mineralization of cementoblasts and periodontal ligament cells. Journal of Periodontology. 2012;**83**(5):672-679. DOI: 10.1902/jop.2011.110408

[26] Rizell S, Kjellberg H, Dietz W, Norén JG, Lundgren T. Altered inorganic composition of dental enamel and dentin in primary teeth from girls with Turner syndrome. European Journal of Oral Sciences. 2010;**118**(2):183-190. DOI: 10.1111/j.1600-0722.2010.00718.x

[27] Veis A. Amelogenin gene splice products: Potential signaling molecules. Cellular and Molecular Life Sciences. 2003;**60**(1):38-55. DOI: 10.1007/s000180300003

[28] Dennis D, Tr AT. Role of amelogenin as predominant organic matrix in enamel biomineralization: Structural and functional aspects. International Journal of Clinical Dentistry. 2018;**11**(3):173-178

[29] Stahl J, Nakano Y, Horst J, Zhu L, Le M, Zhang Y, et al. Exon4 amelogenin transcripts in enamel biomineralization. Journal of Dental Research. 2015;**94**(6):836-842

[30] Galluccio G, Castellano M, La Monaca C. Genetic basis of non-syndromic anomalies of human tooth number. Archives of Oral Biology. 2012;**57**(7):918-930. DOI: 10.1016/j.archoralbio.2012.01.005

[31] Vignesh V, Babu NA, Balachander N, Malathi L. Genes in tooth development. Biomedical & Pharmacology Journal. 2015;**8**(Spl. Edn.):133-138

[32] Ogawa T, Kapadia H, Feng JQ, Raghow R, Peters H, D'Souza RN. Functional consequences of interactions between Pax9 and Msx1 genes in normal and abnormal tooth development. The Journal of Biological Chemistry. 2006;**281**(27):18363-18369. DOI: 10.1074/jbc.M601543200

[33] Kapadia H, Mues G, D'Souza R. Genes affecting tooth morphogenesis. Orthodontics & Craniofacial Research. 2007;**10**(4):237-244. DOI: 10.1111/j.1601-6343.2007.00407.x

[34] Gao Y, Kobayashi H, Ganss B. The human KROX-26/ZNF22 gene is expressed at sites of tooth formation and maps to the locus for permanent tooth agenesis (He-Zhao deficiency). Journal of Dental Research. 2003;**82**(12):1002-1007. DOI: 10.1177/154405910308201213

[35] Al-Batayneh OB. Tricho-dento-osseous syndrome: Diagnosis and dental management. International Journal of Dentistry. 2012;**2012**:514692. DOI: 10.1155/2012/514692

[36] Cobourne MT. Familial human hypodontia—is it all in the genes? British Dental Journal. 2007;**203**(4): 203-208. DOI: 10.1038/bdj.2007.732

[37] Davideau JL, Demri P, Hotton D, Gu TT, MacDougall M, Sharpe P, et al. Comparative study of MSX-2, DLX-5, and DLX-7 gene expression during early human tooth development. Pediatric Research. 1999;**46**(6):650-656

[38] Ortega RM, Requejo AM, Encinas Sotillos A, Andrés P, López-Sobaler AM, Quintas E. Implication of calcium deficiency in the progress of periodontal diseases and osteoporosis. Nutrición Hospitalaria. 1998;**13**(6):316-319

[39] Chen J, Zhang Y, Mendoza J, Denbesten P. Calcium-mediated differentiation of ameloblast lineage cells in vitro. Journal of Experimental Zoology. Part B, Molecular and Developmental Evolution. 2009;**312B**(5):458-464. DOI: 10.1002/jez.b.21279

[40] Nemoto E, Koshikawa Y, Kanaya S, Tsuchiya M, Masato Tamura M, Somerman MJ, et al. Wnt signaling inhibits cementoblast differentiation and promotes proliferation. Bone. 2009;**44**(5):805-812. DOI: 10.1016/j.bone.2008.12.029

[41] Kanaya S, Nemoto E, Ebe Y, Somerman MJ, Shimauchi H. Elevated extracellular calcium increases fibroblast growth factor-2 gene and protein expression levels via a cAMP/PKA dependent pathway in cementoblasts. Bone. 2010;**47**(3):564-572. DOI: 10.1016/j.bone.2010.05.042

[42] Mathias RS, Mathews CH, Machule C, Gao D, Li W, Denbesten PK. Identification of the calcium-sensing receptor in the developing tooth organ. Journal of Bone and Mineral Research. 2001;**16**(12):2238-2244

[43] Spurr NK. Genetics of calcium-sensing—regulation of calcium levels in the body. Current Opinion in Pharmacology. 2003;**3**(3):291-294

[44] Kunert M, Lukomska-Szymanska M. Bio-inductive materials in direct and indirect pulp capping—a review article. Materials. 2020;**13**(5):1204. DOI: 10.3390/ma13051204

[45] Du R, Wu T, Liu W, Li L, Jiang L, Peng W, et al. Role of the extracellular signal-regulated kinase 1/2 pathway in driving tricalcium silicate-induced proliferation and biomineralization of human dental pulp cells in vitro. Journal of Endodontia. 2013;**39**(8):1023-1029. DOI: 10.1016/j.joen.2013.03.002

[46] Okiji T, Yoshiba K. Reparative dentinogenesis induced by mineral trioxide aggregate: A review from the biological and physicochemical points of view. International Journal of Dentistry. 2009;**2009**:464280. DOI: 10.1155/2009/464280

[47] Maeda H, Nakano T, Tomokiyo A, Fujii S, Wada N, Monnouchi S, et al. Mineral trioxide aggregate induces bone morphogenetic protein-2 expression and calcification in human periodontal ligament cells. Journal of Endodontia.

2010;**36**(4):647-652. DOI: 10.1016/j.joen.2009.12.024

[48] Couble ML, Farges JC, Bleicher F, Perrat-Mabillon B, Boudeulle M, Magloire H. Odontoblast differentiation of human dental pulp cells in explant cultures. Calcified Tissue International. 2000;**66**(2):129-138

[49] Kang, KJ., Ryu, CJ. & Jang, YJ. Identification of dentinogenic cell-specific surface antigens in odontoblast-like cells derived from adult dental pulp. Stem Cell Research & Therapy. 2019; 10:128. DOI:org/10.1186/s13287-019-1232-y

[50] Pang L, Zhi Q, Zhuang P, Yu L, Tao Y, Lin H. Variation in namel formation genes influences enamel demineralization *in vitro* in a *Streptococcus mutans* biofilm model. Frontiers in Physiology. 2017;**8**:851. DOI: 10.3389/fphys.2017.00851

[51] Halusic AM, Sepich VR, Shirley DC, Granjeiro JM, Costa MC, Küchler EC, et al. Calcium and magnesium levels in primary tooth enamel and genetic variation in enamel formation genes. Pediatric Dentistry. 2014;**36**(5):384-388

[52] Kumar BS, Priyadarsini KI. Review—selenium nutrition: How important is it? Biomedicine & Preventive Nutrition. 2014;**4**(2):333-341

[53] Pärkö A. Has the increase in selenium intake led to a decrease in caries among children and the young in Finland. Proceedings of the Finnish Dental Society. 1992;**88**(1-2):57-59

[54] Espaladori, MC, Diniz, JMB, de Brito, LCN et al. Selenium intracanal dressing: Effects on the periapical immune response. Clinical Oral Investigations, 2021;**25**:2951-2958. DOI:org/10.1007/s00784-020-03615-8

[55] Codrea CI, Croitoru AM, Baciu CC, Melinescu A, Ficai D, Fruth V, et al. Advances in osteoporotic bone tissue engineering. Journal of Clinical Medicine. 2021;**10**(2):253. DOI: 10.3390/jcm10020253

[56] Römer P, Behr M, Proff P, Faltermeier A, Reicheneder C. Effect of strontium on human Runx2+/− osteoblasts from a patient with cleidocranial dysplasia. European Journal of Pharmacology. 2011;**654**(3):195-199. DOI: 10.1016/j.ejphar.2010.12.031

[57] Huang M, Hill RG, Rawlinson SC. Strontium (Sr) elicits odontogenic differentiation of human dental pulp stem cells (hDPSCs): A therapeutic role for Sr in dentine repair? Acta Biomaterialia. 2016;**38**:201-211. DOI: 10.1016/j.actbio.2016.04.037

[58] Su WT, Wu PS, Ko CS, Huang TY. Osteogenic differentiation and mineralization of human exfoliated deciduous teeth stem cells on modified chitosan scaffold. Materials Science and Engineering C: Materials for Biological Applications. 2014;**41**:152-160. DOI: 10.1016/j.msec.2014.04.048

[59] Tian A, Zhai JJ, Peng Y, Zhang L, Teng MH, Liao J, et al. Osteoblast response to titanium surfaces coated with strontium ranelate-loaded chitosan film. International Journal of Oral & Maxillofacial Implants. 2014;**29**(6):1446-1453. DOI: 10.11607/jomi.3806

[60] Marya CM, Dhingra C. Effect of osteoporosis on oral health. Archives of Medicine. 2015;**8**:2

[61] Jia X, Miron RJ, Yin C, Xu H, Luo T, Wang J, et al. HnRNPL inhibits the osteogenic differentiation of PDLCs stimulated by $SrCl_2$ through repressing Setd2. Journal of Cellular and Molecular Medicine. 2019;**23**(4):2667-2677. DOI: 10.1111/jcmm.14166

[62] Jiang N, Guo W, Chen M, et al. Periodontal ligament and alveolar bone in health and adaptation: Tooth

movement. Frontiers of Oral Biology. 2016;**18**:1-8. DOI: 10.1159/000351894

[63] Hou J, Yamada S, Kajikawa T, Ozaki N, Awata T, Yamaba S, et al. Iron plays a key role in the cytodifferentiation of human periodontal ligament cells. Journal of Periodontal Research. 2014;**49**(2):260-267. DOI: 10.1111/jre.12103

[64] Son, YB., Kang, YH., Lee, HJ. et al. Evaluation of odonto/osteogenic differentiation potential from different regions derived dental tissue stem cells and effect of 17β-estradiol on efficiency. BMC Oral Health. 2021;**21**:15. DOI:org/10.1186/s12903-020-01366-2

[65] Wang L, Yan M, Wang Y, Lei G, Yu Y, Zhao C, et al. Proliferation and osteo/odontoblastic differentiation of stem cells from dental apical papilla in mineralization-inducing medium containing additional KH_2PO_4. Cell Proliferation. 2013;**46**(2):214-222. DOI: 10.1111/cpr.12016

[66] Millán JL, Whyte MP. Alkaline phosphatase and hypophosphatasia. Calcified Tissue International. 2016;**98**:398-416. DOI: 10.1007/s00223-015-0079-1

[67] Rodrigues TL, Foster BL, Silverio KG, Martins L, Casati MZ, Sallum EA, et al. Hypophosphatasia-associated deficiencies in mineralization and gene expression inultured dental pulp cells obtained from human teeth. Journal of Endodontia. 2012;**8**(7):907-912. DOI: 10.1016/j.joen.2012.02.008

[68] Zhu W, Liang M. Periodontal ligament stem cells: Current status, concerns, and future prospects. Stem Cells International. 2015;**2015**:972313. DOI: 10.1155/2015/972313

[69] Heo YY, Um S, Kim SK, Park JM, Seo BM. Responses of periodontal ligament stem cells on various titanium surfaces. Oral Diseases. 2011;**17**(3):320-327. DOI: 10.1111/j.1601-0825.2010.01728.x

[70] Garbo C, Locs J, D'Este M, Demazeau G, Mocanu A, Roman C, et al. Advanced Mg, Zn, Sr, Si multi-substituted hydroxyapatites for bone regeneration. International Journal of Nanomedicine. 2020;**15**:1037-1058. DOI: 10.2147/IJN.S226630

[71] Zhou H, Liang B, Jiang H, Deng Z, Yu K. Magnesium-based biomaterials as emerging agents for bone repair and regeneration: From mechanism to application. Journal of Magnesium and Alloys. 2021;**9**(3):779-804. DOI: org/10.1016/j.jma.2021.03.004

[72] Huang TY, Su WT, Chen PH. Comparing the effects of chitosan scaffolds containing various divalent metal phosphates on osteogenic differentiation of stem cells from human exfoliated deciduous teeth. Biological Trace Element Research. 2018;**185**(2):316-326. DOI: 10.1007/s12011-018-1256-7

[73] Kong Y, Hu X, Zhong Y, Xu K, Wu B, Zheng J. Magnesium-enriched microenvironment promotes odontogenic differentiation in human dental pulp stem cells by activating ERK/BMP2/Smads signaling. Stem Cell Research & Therapy. 2019;**10**(1):378. DOI: 10.1186/s13287-019-1493-5

[74] Anastasiou AD, Nerantzaki M, Gounari E, Duggal MS, Giannoudis PV, Jha A, et al. Antibacterial properties and regenerative potential of Sr^{2+} and Ce^{3+} doped fluorapatites: A potential solution for peri-implantitis. Scientific Reports. 2019;**9**(1):14469. DOI: 10.1038/s41598-019-50916-4

[75] Tsanidou E, Nena E, Rossos A, et al. Caries prevalence and manganese and iron levels of drinking water in school children living in a rural/semi-urban region of North-Eastern Greece. Environmental Health and Preventive

Medicine. 2015;**20**(6):404-409. DOI: 10.1007/s12199-015-0482-2

[76] Arirachakaran P, Benjavongkulchai E, Luengpailin S, Ajdić D, Banas JA. Manganese affects *Streptococcus mutans* virulence gene expression. Caries Research. 2007;**41**(6):503-511

[77] Pizzorno L. Nothing boring about boron. Integrative Medicine. 2015;**14**(4):35-48

[78] Taşlı PN, Doğan A, Demirci S, Şahin F. Boron enhances odontogenic and osteogenic differentiation of human tooth germ stem cells (hTGSCs) in vitro. Biological Trace Element Research. 2013;**53**(1-3):419-427. DOI: 10.1007/s12011-013-9657-0

[79] Nagaraj G, Sukumar A. Evaluation of drinking water trace elements for human health risk assessment. Journal of Ecotoxicology and Environmental Monitoring. 2008;**18**(3):201-215

[80] Nagaraj G, Sukumar A, Nandlal B, Vellaichamy S, Thanasekaran K, AL R. Tooth element levels indicating exposure profiles in diabetic and hypertensive subjects from Mysore, India. Biological Trace Element Research. 2009;**131**:255-262

[81] Thaweboon S, Chunhabundit P, Surarit R, Swasdison S, Suppukpatana P. Effects of lead on the proliferation, protein production, and osteocalcin secretion of human dental pulp cells in vitro. The Southeast Asian Journal of Tropical Medicine and Public Health. 2002;**33**(3):654-661

[82] Abdullah M, Rahman FA, Gnanasegaran N, Govindasamy V, Abu Kasim NH, Musa S. Diverse effects of lead nitrate on the proliferation, differentiation, and gene expression of stem cells isolated from a dental origin. The Scientific World Journal. 2014;**2014**:235941

[83] Irshad M, Scheres N, Crielaard W, Loos BG, Wismeijer D, Laine ML. Influence of titanium on in vitro fibroblast-*Porphyromonas gingivalis* interaction in peri-implantitis. Journal of Clinical Periodontology. 2013;**40**(9):841-849. DOI: 10.1111/jcpe.12136

[84] Wang ML, Nesti LJ, Tuli R, Lazatin J, Danielson KG, Sharkey PF, et al. Titanium particles suppress expression of osteoblastic phenotype in human mesenchymal stem cells. Journal of Orthopaedic Research. 2002;**20**(6):1175-1184. DOI: 10.1016/S0736-0266(02)00076-1

[85] Salvi GE, Bosshardt DD, Lang NP, Abrahamsson I, Berglundh T, Lindhe J, et al. Temporal sequence of hard and soft tissue healing around titanium dental implants. Periodontology 2000. 2015;**68**(1):135-152. DOI: 10.1111/prd.12054

[86] Daubert DM, Pozhitkov AE, Safioti LM, Kotsakis GA. Association of global DNA methylation to titanium and peri-implantitis: A case-control study. JDR Clinical and Translational Research. 2019;**4**(3):284-291. DOI: 10.1177/2380084418822831

[87] Kim, KT, Eo, MY, Nguyen, TTH et al. General review of titanium toxicity. International Journal of Implant Dentistry. 2019;**5**:10. DOI:org/10.1186/s40729-019-0162-x

[88] Zhang X, Wei LC, Wu B, Yu LY, Wang XP, Liu Y. A comparative analysis of metal allergens associated with dental alloy prostheses and the expression of HLA-DR in gingival tissue. Molecular Medicine Reports. 2016;**13**(1):91-98. DOI: 10.3892/mmr.2015.4562

[89] Nakasone Y, Kumagai K, Matsubara R, Shigematsu H, Kitaura K, Suzuki S, et al. Characterization of T cell receptors in a novel murine model of nickel-induced intraoral metal contact allergy. PLoS One. 2018;**13**(12):e0209248. DOI: 10.1371/journal.pone.0209248

[90] Wylie CM, Davenport AJ, Cooper PR, Shelton RM. Oral keratinocyte responses to nickel-based dental casting alloys in vitro. Journal of Biomaterials Applications. 2010;**25**(3):251-267. DOI: 10.1177/0885328209349870

[91] Li L, Drury JL, Zhang H, Sun J, DiJulio D, Chung WO, et al. Effect of Ni(II) on inflammatory gene expression in THP1 monocytic cells. Journal of Biomedical Materials Research. Part A. 2013;**101**(3):902-908. DOI: 10.1002/jbm.a.34369

[92] Messer RL, Lucas LC. Cytotoxicity of nickel-chromium alloys: Bulk alloys compared to multiple ion salt solutions. Dental Materials. 2000;**16**(3):207-212. DOI: 10.1016/s0109-5641(00)00010-5

[93] Rizova H, Carayon P, Barbier A, Lacheretz F, Dubertret L, Michel L. Contact allergens, but not irritants, alter receptor-mediated endocytosis by human epidermal Langerhans cells. British Journal of Dermatology. 1999;**140**(2):200-209

[94] Mao Z, Shay B, Hekmati M, Fermon E, Taylor A, Dafni L, et al. The human tuftelin gene: Cloning and characterization. Gene. 2001;**279**(2): 181-196. DOI: 10.1016/s0378-1119(01)00749-1

[95] Deutsch D, Leiser Y, Shay B, Fermon E, Taylor A, Rosenfeld E, et al. The human tuftelin gene and the expression of tuftelin in mineralizing and nonmineralizing tissues. Connective Tissue Research. 2002;**43**(2-3):425-434. DOI: 10.1080/03008200290001186

[96] Jeremias F, Koruyucu M, Küchler EC, Bayram M, Tuna EB, et al. Genes expressed in dental enamel development are associated with molar-incisor hypomineralization. Archives of Oral Biology. 2013;**58**(10):1434-1442. DOI: 10.1016/j.archoralbio.2013.05.005

Chapter 6

Gene and Cell Therapy in Dental Tissue Regeneration

Juan Andrés de Pablo, Luis Javier Serrano,
Mariano García-Arranz, Luis Romeu and Antonio Liras

Abstract

Advanced therapies hold substantial promise for the treatment of periodontal conditions. Gene therapy has the potential to transfer "therapeutic" genes, which express proteins such as bone morphogenetic proteins, osteoprotegerin, and tissue nonspecific alkaline phosphatase, which is deficient in patients with hypophosphatasia, a condition that affects mineralization of teeth and bone. Transferred genes may also express platelet-derived growth factor, which modulates the growth of periodontal tissue and the alveolar bone. As regards cell therapy, several clinical trials have shown that mesenchymal stem cells, when used with different kinds of scaffolds to enable the required three-dimensional environment, possess a bone regeneration potential that is particularly useful in such disorders as osteoporosis and osteonecrosis, or for regenerating alveolar bone (osseointegration) prior to placing a dental implant. However, much work is still required before these new therapies become true alternatives in routine clinical dental practice. Medical advances require investments, which are usually influenced by the priorities of both politicians and society at large. This will contribute to promoting innovation, efficient treatments, medium- and long-term savings, and a higher quality of life.

Keywords: Advanced therapies, gene therapy, cell therapy, tissue regeneration, alveolar bone, mesenchymal stem cells, biomaterials and scaffolds, implants, Good Manufacturing Practices, clinical dental practice

1. Introduction

Advanced therapies encompass a group of novel and innovative pharmacological procedures including gene therapy, cell therapy and regenerative medicine. Their goal is to provide curative treatment for diseases or dysfunctions that can currently be managed only with palliative care. According to the European Medicines Agency (EMA), advanced therapies are medicines for human use that are based on genes, tissues, or cells, offering ground-breaking new opportunities for the treatment of various diseases of different aetiologies, ranging from hereditary to acquired, such as pathogen-induced infections or cancer [1].

Gene-based medications and procedures are based on "therapeutic" genes whose effect may be curative, but also prophylactic or even diagnostic. By using different transfection methods, advanced therapies aim to insert "recombinant" genes into a diseased cell or organism in order to replace or repair defective genes [2, 3].

Cell therapy procedures involve any cells that no not have the potential to contribute to the genetic material of the subject's offspring (germ-line cells). After minimal manipulation, the cells are "implanted" "or transplanted" autologously (same individual), allogeneically (different individual of the same species) or xenogeneically (individual of a different species) into an organism in order to restore a diseased structure or an impaired function [4, 5].

Regenerative medicine or tissue engineering, for its part, is based on restoring function through the transplantation of cells, tissues, or organoids [6, 7]. Although regenerative medicine procedures are at the present time still at the early stages of development, very promising results have so far been obtained, particularly with regard to organoid preparation [8, 9].

For bioethical reasons, gene therapy procedures are always performed with somatic cells through the transfer of the "therapeutic" gene using viral or non-viral vectors. Transfection efficacy tends to be higher with viral vectors (adeno-associated or lentiviral viruses) but the risk of adverse events is higher, particularly mutagenic insertion, anaphylactic reaction, and hepatotoxic damage. Given that no such thing as an ideal vector exists, a compromise must be struck between sustained long-term expression of the transgene, which entails viral integration of the host cell into the genome, and a reduction in the number of adverse events [10–12].

Gene therapy procedures can be carried out *in vivo* through systemic perfusion of the gene delivery vector, or through *ex-vivo* vector-mediated transfection and subsequent reimplantation of the patient's cells. The latter is an example of the administration of gene therapy followed by cell therapy.

Another more recent alternative is gene editing, which is based on the correction of the defective genes responsible for the patients' symptoms. This technique uses tools such as Talen, zinc fingers or CRISPR/Cas9 gene editing [13].

Other kinds of gene therapy are based on siRNA, whose function is to block RNA translation to protein by temporarily "silencing" a specific gene [14] (**Figure 1**).

As regards the other component of these types of procedures, i.e., the target cells, there is a wide range of possibilities, from pluripotent cells like induced pluripotent stem cells (iPSCs) or embryonic stem cells (ESCs), to multipotent cells, mesenchymal stem cells derived from adipose tissue, bone marrow, umbilical cord, or dental tissue, and differentiated adult cells [15–17].

iPSCs and ESCs are pluripotent cells that must be used with great caution due to their teratogenicity and genetic instability [18]. Use of ESCs is moreover associated with important bioethical issues [19].

Mesenchymal stem cells (MSCs) are currently the only stem cells that have not only shown themselves to be safe in several clinical trials but have also demonstrated their efficacy in a phase III clinical trial, which resulted in their use being approved by the EMA [20] for the treatment of Duchenne muscular dystrophy [21].

Although the mechanism of action of MSCs is not yet fully understood, they are believed to play a role in the process of tissue repair and regeneration, mainly due to their ability to migrate toward damaged or swollen tissues, their angiogenic capacity, their anti-infectious properties and, above all, their immunomodulating and anti-inflammatory effect resulting from the secretion of trophic factors. Moreover, they are responsible for the activation of stem cells that reside in the body and for attracting endogenous cells to the defect site.

Although it is true that one of the most promising options arising from murine models was the use of preconditioned mesenchymal stem cells with different bone morphogenic proteins, unfortunately the *in-vivo* studies performed with larger mammals and the *in-vitro* studies with human mesenchymal cells yielded disappointing results. This prompted the development of fresh research projects, dealing

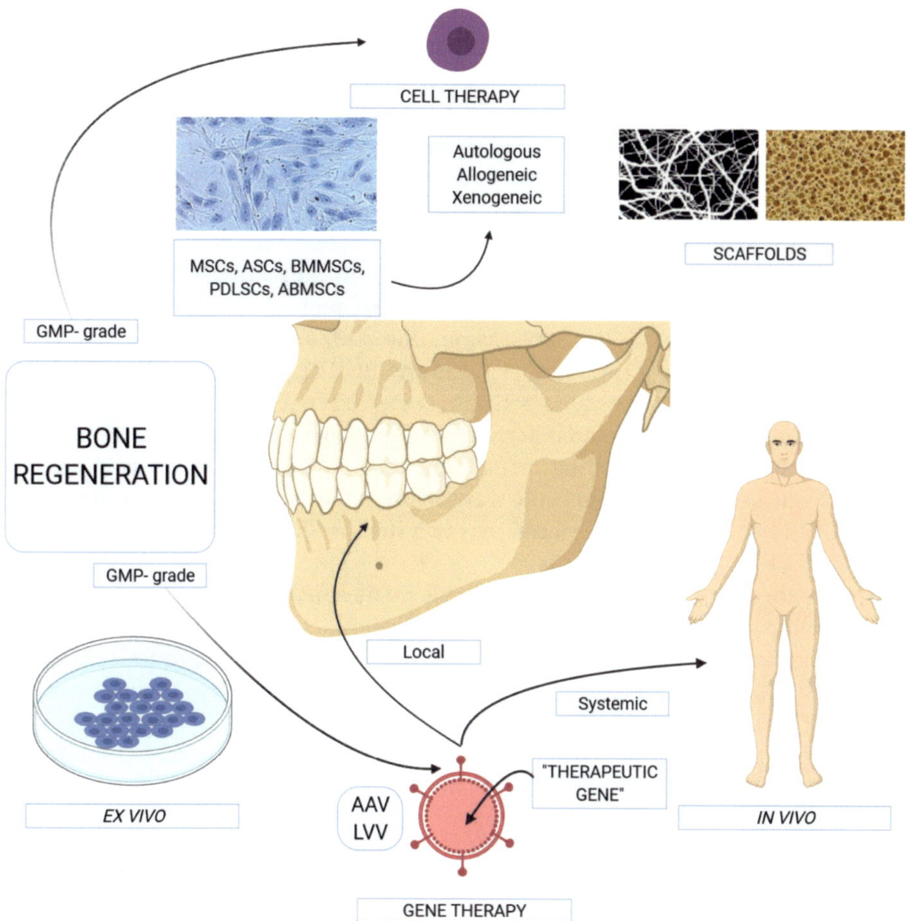

Figure 1.
Application of gene- and cell therapy to bone regeneration. GMP-grade: Good manufacturing practices-grade; MSCs: Mesenchymal stem cells; ASCs: Adipose-derived stem cells; BMMSCs: Bone marrow mesenchymal stem cells; PDLSCs: Periodontal ligament stem cells; ABMSCs: Alveolar bone-derived mesenchymal stem cells; AAV: Adeno-associated viral vectors; LVV: Lentiviral vectors. Cell therapy is one of the techniques used in bone regeneration. MSCs, ASCs, BMMSCs, PDLSCs and autologous, allogenic or xenogenic ABMSCs are used together with scaffolds. Gene therapy procedures can be carried out in vivo through systemic perfusion of the gene delivery vector (AVV, LVV), or through ex-vivo vector-mediated transfection and subsequent reimplantation of the patient's cells. (created in Biorender.com).

particularly with the use of biomaterials to control the ability of MSCs to differentiate and secrete trophic factors by generating a more favorable microenvironment. In the case of a large animal model, the induction of periodontal regeneration through the administration of locally applied growth/differentiation factors is being investigated in non-human primates. Dog models have been developed to study the application of different cells, biomaterials, and scaffolds to periodontal regeneration [22]. In addition, gene therapy protocols based on the transfection of stem cells with viral vectors have been used in mammal models to increase the expression of growth factors [23].

These cells may be isolated from different tissues such as the bone marrow, fat, the umbilical cord, dental pulp, and more recently from endometrium and menstrual blood [16, 24]. They are associated with high proliferation and self-renewal rates, they are capable of secreting countless growth factors, they are easy to obtain and characterize and, most importantly, they are capable of modulating the immune response (they have very low immunogenicity) due to the fact that they express immunomodulating cytokines and do not express the class II major histocompatibility complex (MHC-II) or T-lymphocyte co-stimulating molecules such as CD40L, CD80 y CD86 [25].

They also display a high potential to differentiate to cells of the three germ layers, mesoderm (differentiation to adipocytes, chondrocytes, osteocytes, muscle cells and cardiac cells), endoderm (differentiation to pulmonary epithelial cells) and ectoderm (differentiation into neural cells). For all these reasons, MSCs hold a bright promise in terms of their clinical application [26, 27].

Their morphology is adherent, fibroblast-like and they express characteristic clusters of differentiation (CD) membrane markers such as CD44, CD90, CD117, CD73, CD29, CD13 and CD105. At the same time, they are negative for hematopoietic markers such as CD34, CD45, CD133 and BCRP1. They are endowed with a 46X(X/Y) karyotype that is stable both timewise and in terms of culture passages as it is able to maintain telomerase activity until passage 10. This turns MSCs into a useful cell therapy vehicle as they are exempt from genetic variability and tumorigenesis. They also express embryonic transcription factors such as Oct-4, Rex1 and GATA-4, but not embryonic stem cell markers such as SSEA-1, SSEA-4, TRA-1-60 and TRA-1-81 [28].

Despite the vast amounts of data available on mesenchymal stromal cells and on the different protocols developed for their expansion, characterization and differentiation, as well as for their manufacturing, good manufacturing practice (GMP) protocols for the process extending from the validation of MSCs to their preparation for clinical use, are still in their infancy [29].

The EMA has since 2007 considered expanded MSCs to be advanced therapy medicinal products (ATMPs) fit for clinical use [1].

Although different GMP protocols have been established concerning the isolation and expansion of MSCs, there is still little understanding of the soundness of the required preclinical protocols and their translation to research programs. In this regard, the International Society for Cellular Therapy (ISCT) has established a series of minimum criteria to define the identity and quality of these cells before they can be categorized as ATMPs [30–33]. Although there is some flexibility depending on the types of clinical trials and the regulations issued by different governments, ISCT's fundamental criteria are related with microbiological assays, endotoxin and mycoplasma testing, feasibility tests, clonogenicity, and purity and functionality analyses.

The criteria generally used to validate the use of MSCs in clinical practice are related with the following: manufacturing approval by an ethics committee and participation of authorized sites; donor selection; isolation and expansion of the cells in accordance with GMPs [clonogenicity tests (fibroblast colony-forming units); flow immunocytometry-based cell characterization; differentiation potential assays]; quality control (microbial testing, mycoplasma and endotoxin detection, karyotyping); and shipment from the manufacturing site to the clinical site where they are due to be used in the conditions required for this ATMP (temperature between 3 and 5°C and delivery time under 24 hours) [29].

2. Gene therapy in periodontal disease

As explained above, and as will be specified below, cell therapy is at present the most potentially useful tool to treat periodontal disease. However, gene therapy protocols can also make important contributions in specific cases.

Gene therapy may allow an increase in the bioavailability of certain growth factors or even some proteins that contribute to promoting the modulation of periodontal tissue, specifically alveolar bone. The cells in the periodontal ligament (PDL) are thus characterized by several protein markers such as type III collagen, osteopontin, bone morphogenetic proteins (BMPs), osteocalcin and bone sialoprotein. Among them, BMP-4 is particularly important for bone growth and bone remodeling as it stimulates the expression of osteopontin, BMP-2 and the mRNA of osteoblast-specific transcription factor CBFA1 in human PDL cells. In this respect, Tsuchiya et al. [34] used a (highly safe) non-viral electroporation-based plasmid delivery technique to overexpress BMP-4. *In vitro* transfected rat PDL cells exhibited production and secretion of the mature form of BMP-4 without any cases of inflammation, degeneration, or necrosis.

Also, *ex-vivo* gene therapy experiments have studied the transfer of the BMP-2 gene using bone marrow-derived mesenchymal stromal cells (BMMSCs), muscle-derived cells, adipose-derived stem cells (ASCs), periodontal ligament stem cells, and fibroblasts, also showing an increase in osteogenic differentiation and mineralization [35].

Another interesting approach that used the same protocols consisted in the *in vivo* transfer of the gene that consistently expresses platelet-derived growth factor PDGF-B locally in the alveolar bone, which has been shown to stimulate the regeneration of the periodontal tissue in bone defects in rat models [36]. Periodontal lesions have been treated with a matrix containing adenovirus as a transfer vector expressing PDGF-B. Results showed higher levels of proliferating cell nuclear antigen, with positive cell staining and strong evidence of bone and cementum regeneration. A quantitative analysis showed a nearly four-fold increase in the volume of the alveolar bone and a six-fold increase in the rate of cementum repair in the areas treated with the vector.

Studies on the use of gene therapy to overexpress some proteins related to bone resorption such as osteoprotegerin [37] have shown that these proteins could constitute potential alternatives for modulating and regulating bone mass in cases of bone weakness; alveolar, mandibular, or maxillary bone osteoporosis; or where the alveolar bone needs to be bolstered prior to tooth implantation. Osteoprotegerin is a protein secreted by osteoblasts and stromal osteogenic stem cells that bears close resemblance with other members of the tumor necrosis factor family. It acts as a decoy receptor for receptor activator nuclear factor kappa-B (RANKL) and indirectly inhibits osteoclast differentiation and activation, reducing bone resorption.

In a rat model of periodontitis-derived alveolar bone resorption, non-viral gene therapy-based transfection using a subperiosteally injected osteoprotegerin gene-expressing plasmid achieved a significant reduction in alveolar bone resorption and an increase in the number of active osteoclasts [37].

More recently, gene therapy protocols are successfully being used to study other disorders that would not at first sight seem to be amenable to these techniques, such as hypophosphatasia.

Hypophosphatasia (HPP) is an uncommon hereditary disorder that affects mainly the mineralization of bones and teeth. HPP is caused by loss of function mutations (up to 388 have been reported) in the ALPL gene (chromosome 1) that expresses tissue-nonspecific alkaline phosphatase (TNALP) [38].

Insufficient levels of TNALP, an enzyme found mainly in bone, liver, and renal cells, result in elevated extracellular concentrations of inorganic pyrophosphate (PPi), pyridoxal 5′-phosphate (PLP), and phosphoethanolamine (PEA). The ensuing increase in the extracellular PPi/inorganic phosphate (Pi) relation acts as an inhibitor of bone mineralization, affecting mainly the hard dental tissue (alveolar bone) and resulting in premature tooth loss [39–41].

In general, justification for research into and subsequent application of new advanced therapies depends on the availability (or lack thereof) of an appropriate, convenient, and safe treatment for a given condition. In the case of HPP, treatment before 2015 consisted in an attempt to mitigate symptoms by controlling calcium and phosphorus levels. Enzyme replacement therapy with asfotase alfa has gained popularity in recent years [42], although the treatment is not always effective.

As regards the new advanced therapies, the first few clinical applications corresponded to cell therapy protocols. In this respect, Cahill et al. [43] were able to correct a severe HPP phenotype by transplanting osteoblasts with high levels of TNALP. Migration of these osteoprogenitors to the affected areas of the bone was successful in converting the disease phenotype from severe to mild.

Cell therapy protocols often produce low levels of the deficient protein and, moreover, such production is systemic. For this reason, it is in many cases inevitable to resort to gene therapy protocols which, apart from allowing higher therapeutic efficacy, exhibit longer-term sustained expression levels. Furthermore, they can be applied locally, e.g., in the periodontal tissue. In this regard, Okawa et al., [44] in an *ex-vivo* gene therapy experiment whereby lentiviral vectors and BMMSCs were used with TNALP-deficient knockout mice, were able to induce alveolar bone and cementum formation in those mice, significantly in the first case and moderately in the second, thus contributing to inhibiting premature tooth exfoliation.

More recent gene therapy studies using adeno-associated vectors have shown greater promise. Following administration of the TNALP-expressing adeno-associated vector scAAV8-TNALP to TNALP-deficient knockout mice, Ikeue et al. [45], were successful in achieving enhanced growth of the mandible, the alveolar bone, and the molar roots, inducing dentoalveolar mineralization and reducing the exfoliation risk. The same authors have optimized the efficacy of the technique thereby facilitating its translation to clinical practice [46].

3. Cell therapy and the regeneration of alveolar bone

The periodontium is a complex organ made up of four mesenchymal components (gingiva, cementum, alveolar bone and the PDL), which constitute a functional unit in charge mainly of anchoring the tooth to the jawbone firmly enough to withstand the masticatory forces, and of regulating homeostasis within the oral cavity [47, 48].

The PDL plays a fundamental structural role as it connects the cementum to the alveolar bone. It is a highly vascularized cellular tissue (fibroblasts and endothelial, epithelial, neural, and undifferentiated mesenchymal cells), made up of thick collagen fibers that are inserted into the external layers of the cementum and of the alveolar bone. Dental tissue-derived mesenchymal stem cells are responsible for maintaining hemostasis across all periodontal tissues as they are capable of differentiating to cementoblasts, which give rise to the deposition of cementum; to osteoblasts, which give rise to the deposition of bone; and to fibroblasts, which foster the formation of new connective tissue [47] (**Figure 2**).

Maintenance and regeneration of alveolar bone and of tooth and implant-supporting structures are based on a balance between bone resorption and bone formation [49], which is controlled by different types of cells, signaling mechanisms, and matrix interactions. Advanced therapies, particularly cell therapy and regenerative medicine, could be considered potential tools capable of restoring that balance in soft and hard tissues, making it possible to treat traumatic, metabolic, or congenital disorders that affect periodontal tissue regeneration [50].

This chapter will succinctly cover the possibilities offered by cell therapy for the treatment of disorders related to the loss and defective regeneration of bone mass such as osteoporosis or osteonecrosis (the former understood as a systemic

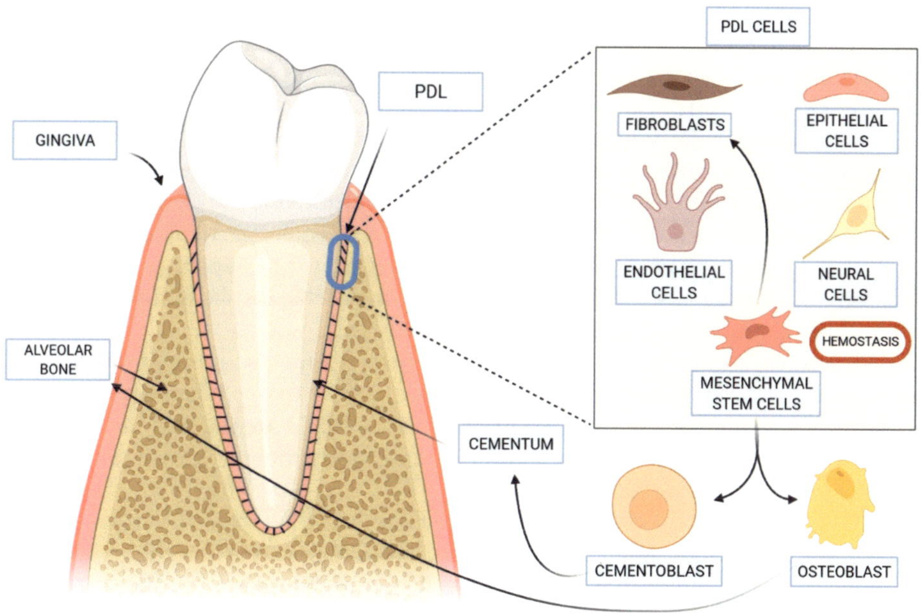

Figure 2.
Periodontium and PDL cells. The periodontium is made up of four mesenchymal components (gingiva, cementum, alveolar bone and the PDL). The PDL, which connects cementum to alveolar bone, is formed by fibroblast, epithelial cells, endothelial cells, neural cells and mesenchymal stem cells. Mesenchymal stem cells are responsible for maintaining bone hemostasis by differentiation to cementoblast, osteoblast and fibroblast. (created in Biorender.com).

metabolic disease of bone and the latter as an apoptotic loss of bone mass, particularly from the alveolar sockets), and for regenerating bone prior to placing a dental implant (osseointegration) [51].

The first pioneering studies on the regeneration of alveolar bone using cell therapy were conducted by Abukawa et al. in 2003 [52]. These authors used porcine MSCs isolated from the bone marrow, which were differentiated to osteoblasts and then incorporated to and cultured on a porous scaffold made from biodegradable poly DL-lactic co-glycolic acid. The result was the formation of bone on the scaffold's surface.

In 2004, the same authors [53] confirmed their results *in vivo* in a porcine model by using autologous constructs (cell-seeded scaffolds) to reconstruct the segmented mandible of the induced model. This resulted in the regeneration of the damaged areas of the mandible, which, in clinical, radiographic, and histologic studies, were found to contain osteoblasts, osteocytes, bone trabeculae and blood vessels.

Some time later, Streckbein et al. [54] marked a turning point in the application of cell therapy to periodontal disease. Indeed, human ASCs became a powerful cell therapy tool. ASCs were found to resemble BMMSCs in their capability of differentiating to osteocytes. Engraftment of autologous ACSs in a fibrin scaffold in a rat model resulted in the formation of significantly greater amounts of bone than in the control group.

3.1 Osteoporosis

Osteoporosis is a chronic (long-term) skeletal condition typically caused by an alteration in bone homeostasis arising from an imbalance between bone resorption and bone formation. Osteoporosis is responsible for the majority of fractures in the elderly and in post-menopausal women, who tend to experience a reduction in bone mass and bone density. Although a genetic predisposition is undeniable, other causative factors such as the slower development of bone mass during youth as well as ethnicity, sex, lifestyle and iatrogenesis usually play a role [55, 56].

Osteoporosis is one of the main causes of alveolar, mandibular, and maxillary bone fractures as these bones are constantly subject to movements and strong masticatory forces, with the mandibular bone withstanding the greatest masticatory forces and exhibiting the most trabecular structure. It is the dentist's job to diagnose potential cases of osteoporosis as early as possible, particularly with a view to evaluating the need of implants. Current treatment for osteoporosis disorder is based on antiresorptive and anabolic drugs (oestrogens, bisphosphonates and monoclonal antibodies such as RANKL inhibitors [55].

What contribution can cell therapy make to the future treatment of this disorder? Simply put, cell therapy can offer "curative" rather than palliative treatment, restoring the structure and function of bone tissue. MSCs are the best candidates on account of their anti-inflammatory and immunologic characteristics, and of their widespread bioethical acceptance [57].

It has been suggested [58] that one of the factors leading to osteoporosis in aged bone tissue is the reduction in the number of MSCs in the bone and the resulting lower osteoblastic differentiation potential. According to several studies, this is where cell therapy would play its most evident clinical role [59–61].

The kind of osteoporosis brought about by post-menopausal estrogen deficiency exhibits very high mortality rates with an associated risk of fracture and of tooth and alveolar bone loss from the jaw. In a study aimed at evaluating the previously stated premise [58] that aging of BMMSCs contributes to the development of osteoporosis, Xu et al. [62] analyzed the effect of special AT-rich sequence-binding protein 2 (SATB2), a regulator of stemness and senescence of craniofacial bone-marrow derived mesenchymal stem cells, on ovariectomy-induced alveolar osteoporosis in a rat model. Transplantation of BMMSCs transfected with the SATB2-expressing gene ameliorated the disease phenotype, reducing cell senescence, increasing stemness and osteogenic capacity, and diminishing the number of osteoclastic markers present as well as the adipogenic potential of the cells and the *in vivo* ovariectomy-induced loss of alveolar bone.

3.2 Osteonecrosis

Osteonecrosis is a clinical entity characterized by apoptosis of the cells that make up the bone and the bone marrow. It is usually associated with the appearance of necrotic areas in the trabecular bone, the subchondral bone, and the bone marrow and, although it could affect any bone, it is most frequently found in the jawbone or, more specifically, the maxilla. Jaw osteonecrosis is an infrequent yet serious condition that involves the maxillary bone [63].

Osteonecrosis generally sets in as a result of exposure of the jawbone to the oral cavity for a period of at least 8 weeks, following which cells (usually osteocytes) become senescent and apoptotic from lack of blood supply from the gingiva. Although there is still no consensus regarding the osteopathogenesis of osteonecrosis, certain situations have been identified as potential causative mechanisms: invasive dental procedures such as tooth extraction surgery; trauma in the area of the maxillary; abnormal (spontaneous) growth of the bone in the palatal area or the internal areas of the mouth, even in patients without identifiable risk factors; radiation therapy (radiation-induced osteonecrosis); head and neck cancer; herpes zoster virus infection; steroid treatments; osteomyelitis; and chronic bone infection. Jaw osteonecrosis may remain asymptomatic for long periods of time, typical symptoms including pain in the affected area, inflammation episodes, redness, and other signs of infection in the gingiva. Patients may experience numbness or a feeling of heaviness in the jaw, develop a purulent secretion in the area of exposed bone, exhibit intra- or extraoral fistulas, or suffer the loosening and loss of the teeth close to the affected area as a result of the weakening of the bone that anchors the teeth [64, 65].

As far as diagnosis is concerned, there is at present no predictive diagnostic test capable of determining if a patient is at risk of or predisposed to suffering jaw osteonecrosis. A number of salivary biomarkers have recently been described, which may potentially help in diagnosing and monitoring the most common oral conditions, including oral leukoplakia, oral lichen planus, Sjögren's syndrome, periodontitis, peri-implantitis, and medication-related osteonecrosis of the jaw [66]. Salivary biomarkers such as interleukins or growth factors have shown themselves useful in diagnosing and following up these conditions, making it possible to conduct an early evaluation of the risk of malignization and monitor the efficacy of treatment.

Treatments based on antiresorptive drugs such as bisphosphonates administered to patients at high risk of osteoporosis or as treatment for bone cancer have often resulted in an increase in jaw osteonecrosis [67, 68]. The mechanism by which bisphosphonates may result in maxillary osteonecrosis are currently not understood, but they have been shown to affect dentoalveolar structures, limiting or impeding bone regeneration due to inhibition of osteoclast formation and/or suppression of cell turnover.

Prevention through health education, dental hygiene and periodic dental visits from early childhood is essential. In most cases, a detailed anamnesis is crucial for both early detection and prevention [69–71]. Routine treatment is based on antibiotics, antibacterial mouthwashes such chlorhexidine, and removable oral appliances (retainers) or dental debridement.

There being currently no standard treatment to promote regeneration of the necrotized area, advanced therapies and, specifically cell therapy, are emerging as valuable tools not only to curb the necrosis but also to restore and regenerate the necrotized areas. Although studies have so far focused on bisphosphonate-induced jaw osteonecrosis, the solutions they propose – if effective – could be applied to most kinds of jaw osteonecrosis, regardless of their etiopathogenesis.

The first clinical trial that used cell therapy to attempt regeneration of the alveolar maxillary bone was conducted in 2009 by d'Aquino et al. [72]. The authors used a biocomplex consisting of autologous dental pulp stem cells and a collagen scaffold. Histological observation unambiguously showed complete regeneration of the bone at the necrotic site with optimal rehabilitation of the alveolar bone and full restoration of the periodontal tissue.

Very good alveolar bone regeneration results have also been obtained in bisphosphonate-induced osteonecrosis models using allogeneic bone marrow [73] or ASCs [74]. The advantage of ASCs, as compared to BMMSCs, lies in their easy and less invasive harvest, their higher yield, their higher proliferation and duplication potential, their lower levels of senescence; and their higher angiogenic anti-inflammatory capacity. These cells also exhibit higher survival rates in ischemic environments as well as an increased secretion of growth factors such as the vascular endothelial growth factor (VEGF), hepatocyte growth factor (HGF), and basic fibroblast growth factor (bFGF). These factors are required in hypoxic environments, which is useful for the treatment of osteonecrosis and bisphosphonate-related ischemic wounds derived from jaw osteonecrosis [74, 75].

There is currently only one clinical trial underway aimed at evaluating the use of cell therapy for the treatment of jaw osteonecrosis [76]. It specifically seeks to determine the safety of using autologous BMMSCs in the presence of a porous tricalcium phosphate scaffold and in a demineralized bone matrix in patients with jaw osteonecrosis. It is a phase I, prospective non-randomized single-centre unblinded open clinical trial including patients between 18 and 85 years of age. The study is the result of a collaborative effort between the Virgen de la Arrixaca Institute of BioHealth Research (Region of Murcia), the Virgen de la Arrixaca University Hospital (Region of Murcia), the Regional Ministry of Health of Murcia and the Spanish Ministry of Health.

Patients with a definitive clinical and radiological diagnosis of jaw osteonecrosis, of whatever etiology, are implanted with the cell "construct" (MSCs, tricalcium phosphate and demineralized bone matrix). One month prior to implantation, the MSCs are first harvested from the patients' bone marrow and then characterized and expanded in GMP-grade conditions. The cells are seeded in tricalcium phosphate and maintained in culture for 14 days. On the day of implantation, the MSCs seeded in tricalcium phosphate are admixed with the demineralized bone matrix, the combination being subsequently coagulated with autologous platelet-rich plasma before engraftment can occur. Finally, the oral mucosa or the skin are closed tightly with silk sutures. A careful evaluation must be made of different circumstances related with the procedure such as bone ischemia or new bone formation; non-severe adverse events related with the procedure such as local surgical wound infections, non-union and anaphylactic reactions; time to wound healing; appearance of local pain as determined by a visual analogue scale; bone formation as measured by computerized tomography; and quality of life as measured by EuroQol-5D [77, 78].

Mesenchymal stem cells could also play an important osteogenesis and bone regeneration role in cases of osteoradionecrosis [79], a severe and difficult-to-manage complication of the jawbone following high-dose radiation therapy in cases of head and neck cancer.

3.3 Bone regeneration and osseointegration prior to dental implant placement

Placement of intraosseous implants is a routine dental procedure aimed at restoring missing teeth and masticatory function. However, the stability of implants is often compromised by the presence of an insufficient amount of supporting bone mass. Sinus elevation treatment using autologous bone and allografts is the standard alternative in these cases. The problem lies in amount of autologous bone required for such procedures, which varies as a function of the magnitude of the damage present. Moreover, alternative alloplastic materials are often ill suited to compromised vascular environments.

Initial studies in this field, such as those by Matsuo et al. [80] have made interesting contributions. Using particulate cellular bone and marrow (PCBM) and platelet-rich plasma (PRP), these authors obtained statistically significant increases in the volume of trabecular bone. Equally interesting findings were reported by Trautvetter et al. [81] who evaluated the effect of applying autologous periosteal bone grafts in conjunction with scaffolds to atrophic maxillary bone on long-term clinical restoration in one-stage procedures, which also involved placement of dental implants. At six months post-op, these authors observed the presence of trabecular bone with active osteocytes and osteoblasts and no signs of bone resorption, connective tissue formation or necrosis.

Different alternatives have been tested, with varying degrees of success in an attempt to achieve bone regeneration, including multiple biomaterials and scaffolds (both natural and artificial), different types of stem cells obtained from the dental follicle, the periodontal ligament, the dental pulp, the salivary glands and the adipose tissue; and the multiple growth factors used for dentistry applications in the framework of tissue engineering programs. Nonetheless, developing new methodologies and strategies is required to address the problems inherent in the reconstruction of periodontal bones and tissues [82].

Further in-depth research will be required to determine the influence of the microenvironment inside the damaged periodontium on the efficacy of the new strategies that are being developed [83]. The microenvironment exerts a very significant influence on physiological and physiopathological function, and on the therapeutic effect of MSCs. The niche where these cells reside is made up of multiple cell populations, tissue components, and soluble factors that regulate the cells' behavior. The fact that viability and differentiation of MSCs are compromised in conditions such as osteoporosis and periodontitis may aggravate the patient's condition and disrupt the tissue healing process.

Studies are currently underway to investigate ways of improving and optimizing the microenvironment where transplanted cells are going to reside. These studies have used either pharmacological or epigenetic techniques [84], or cell-free (extracellular vesicle-based) applications [85] to enhance the resistance of exogenous MSCs.

In any event, whether by classical methods or by cell therapy protocols, all efforts should be aimed at achieving osseointegration to enhance implant efficiency and durability [86]. The key milestones on the road to osseointegration are as follows: firstly, it is essential to make sure that periodontal tissue responds positively to the implant from the outset; subsequently, it must induce osteogenesis and bone remodeling around the implant. As osseointegration is a process mediated by the innate immune system that involves the complement system and reactive macrophages, factors such as the design and the chemical composition of the implant, the surgical technique employed, the use of "therapeutic cells", the local microenvironment and the patient's systemic characteristics, may play a significant role.

Recourse to StemBios Cell therapy has facilitated induction of early osseointegration in primary dental implants. StemBios Cells® are pluripotent stem cells derived from adult blood and bone marrow. They are equipped with specific biomarkers and can be easily cultured *in vitro* in large quantities. They possess the advantages of embryonic stem cells but, unlike them, they are not teratogenic, and they cannot result in immunologic rejection. They are capable of differentiating to endodermal, mesodermal and ectodermal cells, both *in vivo* and *in vitro*. In an analysis of 11 subjects who had received a dental implant in the mandible only one of whom was treated with StemBios cell therapy at the time of implantation, Weng et al. [87] found that this subject exhibited superior healing of the bone tissue, particularly regarding early bone ingrowth, as compared with that observed following implantation without this kind of cell therapy.

More recently [88] it has been shown that BMMSCs play an important role in the efficacy and induction of osseointegration following dental implant placement. Uncontrolled diabetes mellitus is known to result in very poor osseointegration and reduced implant durability. Alqahtani et al. analyzed the effect of BMMSCs in the presence of platelet-rich plasma on the osseointegration of implants placed in New Zealand rabbits with induced type 1 diabetes. Implants were placed with the help of collagen sponges loaded with osteoinductive BMMSCs and platelet-rich plasma. Osseointegration was significantly more effective in the presence of BMMSCs than in implantations where only platelet-rich plasma was used.

As other tissues in the human body, periodontal tissues are endowed with a reservoir of MSCs that share the same characteristics as other mesenchymal cells such as adherence, the potential to differentiate to at least three cell lines, and specific cluster of differentiation markers for stromal cells [89]. In addition, these cells possess immunomodulating functions. Their properties make these cells potentially applicable in clinical practice for the treatment of periodontal and other conditions, even neurodegenerative ones, such as Parkinson's disease [90].

The first mesenchymal cells isolated from periodontal tissues were human dental pulp stem cells (hDPSCs), followed by apical papilla stem cells (SCAPs), periodontal ligament stem cells (PDLSCs), gingiva-derived mesenchymal stem cells (GMSCs), dental follicle stem cells (DFSCs), tooth germ stem cells (TGSCs), and alveolar bone-derived mesenchymal stem cells (ABMSCs). PDLSCs, GMSCs, TGSCs, SCAPs and ABMSCs, the latter sharing many characteristics with BMMSCs, present osteogenic capacity. For their part, DFSCs play a role in the formation of alveolar bone and the root-bone interface in tooth development [89].

Unfortunately, the number of stromal cells that can be obtained from periodontal tissue is extremely low, which represents a significant hurdle for the use of those cells when harvested autologously (directly from the patient). This makes it necessary to use other allogeneic sources of adult tissue such as BMMSCs and, especially, ASCs, given their greater ease of harvest and greater yield [91].

As a general concept cell therapy, as used to regenerate periodontal bone tissue, is based on a combination of a cellular element, made up of the patient's own autologous mesenchymal stem cells, an extracellular element, or scaffold, that provides a substrate for tissue growth and, lastly, a series of chemical-molecular elements, mainly trophic and growth factors secreted by the cells themselves, that play a role in the regenerative process. In other words, cell therapy involves an osteogenic cellular component, a series of osteoconductive signals (trophic factors) and an osteoconductive support component (scaffold). In this regard, given that there are multiple factors that may have an impact on the success of these new therapies, the results of translating the findings of preclinical trials using *in vivo* animal models to the human clinical setting, are not always the ones initially expected. The reasons for this discrepancy are basically related with size-related differences between human and animal defects and with what is known as "diffusion distances," which have to do with limitations to massive transport (e.g., oxygen diffusion and elimination of metabolic waste), which are essential for the survival of the transplanted cells. Moreover, as mentioned above, there may exist significant differences between animal and human models in terms of the local microenvironment where the cells reside, and in terms of the epigenetic processes at work in each of them. These aspects are likely to exert a huge impact on the results obtained [83, 84]. For these reasons, hystomorphometric analysis of biopsy samples is the most effective way of quantitatively evaluating regeneration of the bone structure [92].

It should be noted that, when applying advanced therapies (MSC-based therapy), apart from measuring the efficacy of the procedure, it is essential to consider its cost-effectiveness. Although the cost involved in the expansion and preparation of cells is high in GMP-grade procedures [29], several studies [93] have confirmed that, taking into account the indirect costs related to hospitalization and complementary treatments such as general anesthesia and the higher complications rate and higher morbidity associated with traditional grafting procedures, the cost-efficiency of the new advanced therapies could be higher.

3.4 Clinical trials in progress

As mentioned above in this chapter, although we have a robust understanding of the properties of stem cells and of the viral vectors used for gene transfer, there still remains work to be done before they can be applied to clinical practice, including GMP protocols [29]. The gap will be bridged gradually as the results of the different clinical trials underway on the new or advanced therapies become available. The ISCT has already established a series of minimal safety requirements that must be met when defining the identity and quality of these cells as ATMPs. These requirements are mainly related with the risk of contamination by pathogens, the presence of endotoxins and mycoplasma, the viability of the cells, the safety of the viral vectors and the teratogenic safety of the cells. These requirements must unfailingly be met by any clinical study that is undertaken.

One of the first successful clinical trials that used BMMSCs was performed by Gjerde et al. (ClinicalTrials.gov *identifier: NCT02751125*) [94, 95], which started enrolling patients in April 2016 and was concluded in March 2020. The trial was sponsored by the University of Bergen with the collaboration of Ulm University, Haukeland University Hospital, University of Nantes, Madrid's Complutense University, the University of Aarhus, the International University of Catalonia, Assistance Publique - Hôpitaux de Paris and the European Commission. It was a pilot project aimed at reconstructing atrophied posterior mandibular alveolar ridges by using biomaterials and autologous BMMSCs. The last step in the process was the insertion of an implant into the newly formed bone. This was an interventional clinical trial with 13 subjects, between 18 and 80 years (**Figure 3**).

Cells were obtained from the bone marrow of the patients' alveolar ridge. The sample was processed in a cell therapy lab using GMP-grade protocols. Cells were expanded and characterized through flow immunocytometry and, 21 days later, they were transplanted to the subjects' alveolar bone. Before closing the transplant site, the cells were brought into contact with dicalcium phosphate (DCP) and the material was covered with a reinforced titanium membrane. From four to six months later, the bone was biopsied and implants placed in the regenerated bone. Patients were followed up for 1, 2, 3 and 5 years to assess the stability of the implant. Moreover, the newly formed bone was clinically and radiologically assessed. Implant stability was measured using the Ostell™ system, based on Resonance Frequency Analysis (RFA) [96]. In addition, an evaluation was made of potential adverse events derived from the treatment in general and of the cells in particular (safety and tolerability).

Results showed that clinical reconstruction of the alveolar ridge is a feasible and safe procedure yielding a predictable outcome. Osseointegration was achieved in all dental implants.

A promising clinical trial (ClinicalTrials.gov *identifier: NCT04297813*) got underway in March 2020. It is meant to be the first controlled trial using autologous mesenchymal stem cells, cultured, expanded, and maintained using synthetic biomaterials with the aim of regenerating enough maxillary bone to offer support to dental implants. The coordinators of the study are Pierre Layrolle, from the University of Nantes (France) and Kamal Mustafa, from the University of Bergen (Norway) and it is sponsored by the European Union (H2020 Maxibone Project). This clinical trial follows on from a previous study by Gjerde et al. [94, 95].

It is a phase III interventional multicentre randomized controlled clinical trial of 150 patients over 18 years of age. It is aimed at comparing the safety and efficacy of using autologous mesenchymal stem cells cultured on calcium phosphate biomaterials against the use of autologous bone grafts. Patients have been randomized into either a control group, where subjects receive standard treatment (a jawbone graft), or an experimental group, where subjects receive a combination of biomaterials and cultured and expanded autologous stem cells [97].

The cells are obtained from the patients' coxal bone marrow. These stem cells are being expanded and produced in two different labs, one at the Transfusional and Immunogenetic Medicine Institute of the University of Ulm (Germany), and the other at the Créteil Centre de Thérapie Cellulaire (France). After two weeks, the mesenchymal stem cells are sent to a surgical clinical centre where they are brought into contact with a biomaterial (DCP) and, subsequently, engrafted onto

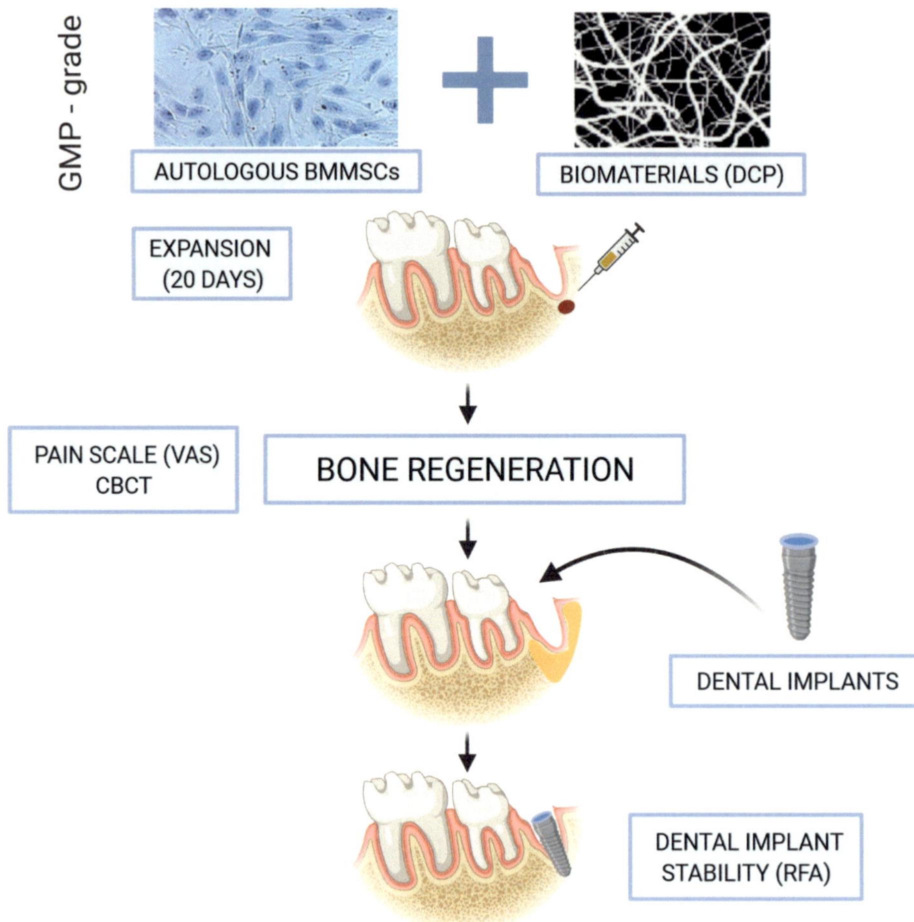

Figure 3.
Clinical trials currently in progress. GMP-grade: good manufacturing practices-grade; BMMSCs: bone marrow mesenchymal stem cells; DCP: dicalcium phosphate; VAS: visual analog scale; CBCT: cone beam computed tomography; RFA: resonance frequency analysis. These clinical trials are based on the use of BMMSCs together with dicalcium phosphate (DCP). The objective was to reconstruct atrophied posterior mandibular alveolar ridges by using biomaterials and autologous BMMSCs. The last step in the process was the insertion of an implant into the newly formed bone. Patients were followed clinically and radiologically. (Created in Biorender.com).

the maxillary and mandibular alveolar ridges. Patients in the control group are engrafted with autologous bone from the posterior mandibular ramus. A non-resorbable membrane is used to cover the grafts and guide the tissue regeneration process. Five months later, the implants are placed following an assessment of the amount of bone regeneration obtained. Bone biopsies are then obtained, which are evaluated by synchrotron, microcomputerised tomography and histology. Subsequently, once dental implants have become osteointegrated, the protective elements can be placed.

The primary outcome measure in this study will be an evaluation of the changes in the linear measurements of the alveolar bone width, as measured below the alveolar ridge immediately before placement of the implant. Secondary outcome measures will consist, on the one hand, in a VAS evaluation of postoperative pain following each of the two treatments [98] and, on the other, of radiological analyses to determine the bone volume present, thus gauging the amount of new bone obtained. This will allow making an informed decision regarding the possibility of placing an implant in the reconstructed area. Such as decision will be made on the basis of 3D Cone Beam Computed Tomography (CBCT) [99].

To be included in the trial subjects have to be healthy, non-smokers and in need of implants in the upper or lower jaw, with loss of vertical height and less than 4 mm lateral width. Exclusion criteria include the general contraindications for dental and/or surgical treatment, and for harvesting bone marrow specimens or bone grafts; a history of any malignant disease; previous or concurrent radiation therapy of the head and neck; a history of infectious diseases (HIV, syphilis, hepatitis B or C); uncontrolled diabetes mellitus; inflammatory or autoimmune diseases of the oral cavity; and previous or concurrent immunosuppressive treatment or high-dose bisphosphonate or corticosteroid therapy.

4. Reflections on the application of advanced therapies in dentistry

Advanced therapies encompass a wide-ranging series of different therapeutic procedures that can be applied to most conditions, transmissible or otherwise [100]. They are multidisciplinary procedures that may involve basic molecular and cellular biology techniques and tissue engineering [101]. In general, implementation of a new healthcare technology, understood in this case as a new therapeutic procedure, has vast repercussions not only from the clinical point of view but also from a social and economic perspective. This places a heavy responsibility on the shoulders of managers and officials in charge of its application. To this should be added human innate reluctance to adopt new ideas especially when, as in the case of the new therapies, there are so many unknowns regarding potential medium and long-term effects. However, some clinical disciplines are more open to change than others. This should be considered together with the social, legal and bioethical considerations associated to the introduction of any new technology [102–104].

An explanation must be found to the fact that despite the significant progress made and the success obtained by research into ATMPs in the last few years, the number of procedures and products authorized by evaluation agencies has been extremely low and limited to relatively severe conditions. Going back to dentistry, although significant improvements have been made on the more classical techniques and on advanced therapies, much work remains to be done before many of these procedures become standard clinical practice. The reasons for this may be related to the novelty of the techniques themselves or to other factors of a social, economic, or bioethical-legal nature, without mentioning the inherent distrust of practitioners and the general public toward these innovative procedures. Indeed, even if dental conditions are not in principle potentially fatal and may often be prevented, they are highly prevalent, affecting more than 3,5 billion people worldwide [105]. They are therefore associated with a high economic cost and, very often, a low quality of life. They are also a social problem as they typically affect the less affluent social classes [106]. Moreover, dental infections could result in a worsening of systemic conditions, such as cardiovascular disease [107, 108]. For all these reasons, any procedure that may ensure greater medium- and long-term efficacy of dental procedures should be eagerly embraced.

What could then be the reasons behind the low number of patients enrolled in advanced therapy programs in routine periodontal practice? The first explanation, applicable to any type of condition except severe or fatal ones, is the lack of a sufficient number of preclinical and clinical trials to confirm the therapy's efficacy and, particularly, its safety. As advanced therapy procedures were introduced only recently, their potential, especially long-term, adverse events are not known. It is therefore essential for a whole body of new clinical trials to be undertaken to dispel misgivings and promote confidence among patients. This will inevitably require greater economic investments in research.

As far as the safety of these protocols is concerned, the more stringent requirements imposed by regulatory agencies typically results in a delay in the implementation of these new therapies. In this regard, special programmes have been introduced in the last few years to accelerate regulatory procedures and overcome the so-called "valley of death," which tends to hold up the deployment of these novel procedures in clinical practice [109–113].

ATMPs are regulated in the European Union by Directives 1394/2007 [114] and 2009/120/EC [115], which amended Directive 2001/83/EC. Those products are controlled by the Committee for Advanced Therapies and the Committee for Medicinal Products for Human Use of the European Medicines Agency (EMA), the European equivalent of the United States' Food and Drug Administration (FDA). The drug regulatory agencies of Australia [116], Canada [117], the United States [118], Korea [119], Singapore [120] and Japan [121] have developed a specific framework for regulating their use [122].

Meeting the requirements for the accreditation, designation, authorization, or licensing of the tissue establishments and cell preparation processes involved in advanced therapy medicinal products can be challenging. As explained above, the main goal is to ensure that such processes are safe. However, it must be considered that regulatory agencies prefer to tread cautiously into this uncharted territory so full of legal loopholes. Apart from addressing those loopholes, which is the responsibility of the legislative bodies, an attempt should be made at harmonizing the safety norms applicable to advanced therapy medicinal products across the different regulatory agencies, particularly concerning their general principles, which seem to be more skewed toward ensuring patient safety than facilitating the development of innovative therapies to address current medical challenges. This is of course complicated by the fact that the handling and manipulation of cells and tissue materials must be performed under Good Manufacturing Practice (GMP) conditions as regulated by Directive 2003/94/EC [123].

It is therefore necessary to find a compromise between the three terms in the equation: safety, economic investments, and cost-efficiency. In severe or fatal conditions cost-efficiency tends to be very high but in others such as dental conditions, which are typically non-fatal, there being other longer-standing and more economical alternatives cost-efficiency is usually much lower. A consensus must be reached between academia, industry, regulatory authorities, and other stakeholders that paves the way to improving the design of ATMPs, facilitating their use, and making it easier for them to make the transition from bench to bedside. In other words, regulation, reimbursement, and realization are the 3 Rs [124] required to ensure that patients can benefit from advanced therapies in a safe and efficient way.

It could be argued that the lack of correlation between novel ideas and therapeutic procedures on the one hand, and clinical practice on the other, is generally due not so much to scientific reasons but rather to regulatory and cost-related ones. It must be considered that advanced therapies are essentially personalized rather than one-size-fits-all therapies, which inevitably leads to higher design and production costs [125].

It should not be forgotten that the rate of progress in a given clinical domain is determined by the importance assigned by governments and societies to advances in that domain. Indeed, implementation of novel technologies is heavily influenced by their usefulness in the eyes of society, particularly in the face of an ever-increasing life expectancy, which inevitable leads to a rise in the number of comorbidities. From a dentistry perspective, dental problems resulting from a longer life expectancy lead to a lower quality of life because of a disturbed masticatory function.

Priorities in the realm of dentistry are also influenced by the idiosyncrasies and the mindsets of the different countries and geographical regions with respect to healthcare policy. In some Western countries, dental care and hygiene have been considered to play a secondary role, which has resulted in a lack of awareness of the importance of dental education and an ensuing lack of prevention programs. Some governments do not seem willing to devote the required resources to address conditions that might not appear excessively severe at first glance, but which result in significant direct and indirect social costs in the medium or long-term.

Implementation of new therapeutic strategies and procedures is clearly constrained by the level of priority given to specific clinical areas, starting at the base of the pyramid, which is prevention-oriented health education. In dentistry, as well as in other areas, it is essential to support research into new therapies based on ATMPs in order to provide patients with alternative dental treatments that are safer and more effective in the long term.

5. Conclusions

- The topic addressed in this chapter, i.e., the contribution of gene and cell therapy to dental tissue regeneration, is closely related to developmental dental defects and their treatment. Protocols based on gene and cell therapy represent "curative" rather than "palliative" therapeutic tools for defects affecting human dental hard tissues. Proteomics, genomics, and biomaterials science will be instrumental for translating these strategies into clinical practice.

- Advanced therapies constitute potentially essential strategies for the treatment of periodontal disease.

- Gene therapy, through adeno-associated or lentiviral vectors could activate periodontal tissue and alveolar bone modulation through the transfer of "therapeutic" genes expressing proteins such as BMPs, osteoprotegerin, or tissue- nonspecific alkaline phosphatase, which is deficient in patients with HPP (a condition that affects mineralization of teeth and bone) among others. Those genes could also express factors such as the platelet-derived growth factor.

- In cell therapy, mesenchymal stem cells implemented in an autologous, allogeneic or xenogeneic manner, with the aid of scaffolds to enable the required three-dimensional environment, have been shown by several clinical trials to have a significant bone regeneration potential in the context of osteoporosis, osteonecrosis or alveolar bone regeneration (osseointegration) prior to placement of a dental implant. Use of these cells is safe as they do not present with teratogenicity, they have immunomodulating properties, and they do not pose the risk of immune rejection. The implanted cells maintain homeostasis across all periodontal tissues and are capable of preserving and regenerating the alveolar bone and the tooth and implant supporting structures by managing the balance between bone formation and bone resorption. The results obtained have thus far offered significant promise in terms of the long-term durability of implants given the efficacy observed in the induction of osseointegration.

- Implementation of the new therapies will require finding a compromise between safety, economic investments, and cost-efficiency. It will be necessary to reach a consensus between academia, industry, and the regulatory authorities to improve the design of ATMPs, facilitate their use and speed up their translation to clinical practice.

- Advanced therapies are by definition personalized, which increases the costs inherent in their design and their production. For that reason, it will be essential going forward to devote greater resources to the clinical areas where they have shown greatest promise. As regards the implementation of advanced therapies in dentistry, it will be necessary to raise people's awareness about the importance of good dental health because as the investments required by medical progress and these are heavily influenced by the priorities of governments and society at large. A greater awareness will contribute to promoting innovation, efficient treatments, medium- and long-term savings, and a higher quality of life.

Conflict of interest

The authors declare no conflict of interest.

Author details

Juan Andrés de Pablo[1], Luis Javier Serrano[1], Mariano García-Arranz[2], Luis Romeu[3] and Antonio Liras[1,2]*

1 Department of Genetics, Physiology, and Microbiology, Complutense University of Madrid, Spain

2 New Therapies Laboratory, Health Research Institute-Fundación Jiménez Díaz University Hospital (IIS-FJD), Madrid, Spain

3 Department of Dentistry, Complutense University of Madrid, Spain

*Address all correspondence to: aliras@ucm.es

References

[1] European Commission. Regulation (EC) No 1394/2007 of the European Parliament and of the Council of 13 November 2007 on advanced therapy medicinal products and amending Directive 2001/ 83/EC and Regulation (EC) No 726/2004. Official Journal of the European Union 2007; 50(1): 121-137.

[2] Anguela XM, High KA. Entering the Modern Era of Gene Therapy. Annu Rev Med 2019; 70: 273-288. DOI: 10.1146/annurev-med-012017-043332.

[3] High KA, Roncarolo MG. Gene Therapy. N Engl J Med 2019; 381(5): 455-464. DOI: 10.1056/NEJMra1706910.

[4] Campbell A, Brieva T, Raviv L, Rowley J, Niss K, Brandwein H, et al. Concise Review: Process Development Considerations for Cell Therapy. Stem Cells Transl Med 2015; 4(10): 1155-1163. DOI: 10.5966/sctm.2014-0294.

[5] Zakrzewski W, Dobrzyński M, Szymonowicz M, Rybak Z. Stem cells: past, present, and future. Stem Cell Res Ther 2019; 10(1): 68. DOI: 10.1186/s13287-019-1165-5.

[6] Witten CM, McFarland RD, Simek SL. Concise Review: The U.S. Food and Drug Administration and Regenerative Medicine. Stem Cells Transl Med 2015; 4(12): 1495-1499. DOI: 10.5966/sctm.2015-0098.

[7] Trohatou O, Roubelakis MG. Mesenchymal Stem/Stromal Cells in Regenerative Medicine: Past, Present, and Future. Cell Reprogram 2017; 19(4): 217-224. DOI: 10.1089/cell.2016.0062.

[8] Li M, Izpisua JC. Organoids: Preclinical Models of Human Disease. N Engl J Med 2019; 380: 569-579. DOI: 10.1056/NEJMra1806175.

[9] Cui H, Nowicki M, Fisher JP, Zhang LG. 3D Bioprinting for Organ Regeneration. Adv Healthc Mater 2017; 6(1): 10.1002/adhm.201601118. DOI: 10.1002/adhm.201601118.

[10] Mendell JR, Al-Zaidy SA, Rodino-Klapac LR, Goodspeed K, Gray SJ, Kay CN, et al. Current Clinical Applications of In Vivo Gene Therapy with AAVs. Mol Ther 2020; S1525-0016(20)30664-X. DOI: 10.1016/j.ymthe.2020.12.007.

[11] Martínez-Molina E, Chocarro-Wrona C, Martínez-Moreno D, Marchal JA, Boulaiz H. Large-Scale Production of Lentiviral Vectors: Current Perspectives and Challenges. Pharmaceutics 2020; 12(11): 1051. DOI: 10.3390/pharmaceutics12111051.

[12] Harris E, Elmer JJ. Optimization of electroporation and other non-viral gene delivery strategies for T cells. Biotechnol Prog 2020; e3066. DOI: 10.1002/btpr.3066.

[13] Janik E, Niemcewicz M, Ceremuga M, Krzowski L, Saluk-Bijak J, Bijak M. Various Aspects of a Gene Editing System-CRISPR-Cas9. Int J Mol Sci 2020; 21(24): 9604. DOI: 10.3390/ijms21249604.

[14] Saw PE, Song EW. siRNA therapeutics: a clinical reality. Sci China Life Sci 2020; 63(4): 485-500. DOI: 10.1007/s11427-018-9438-y.

[15] Doss MX, Sachinidis A. Current Challenges of iPSC-Based Disease Modeling and Therapeutic Implications. Cells 2019; 8(5): 403. DOI: 10.3390/cells8050403.

[16] Berebichez-Fridman R, Montero-Olvera PR. Sources and Clinical Applications of Mesenchymal Stem Cells: State-of-the-art review. Sultan Qaboos Univ Med J 2018; 18(3): e264-e277. DOI: 10.18295/squmj.2018.18.03.002.

[17] Baniebrahimi G, Khanmo hammadi R, Mir F. Teeth-derived stem cells: A source for cell therapy. J Cell Physiol 2019; 234(3): 2426-2435. DOI: 10.1002/jcp.27270.

[18] Shinde V, Sureshkumar P, Sotiriadou I, Hescheler J, Sachinidis A. Human Embryonic and Induced Pluripotent Stem Cell Based Toxicity Testing Models: Future Applications in New Drug Discovery. Curr Med Chem 2016; 23(30): 3495-3509. DOI: 10.2174/0929867323666160627113436.

[19] King NM, Perrin J. Ethical issues in stem cell research and therapy. Stem Cell Res Ther 2014; 5(4): 85. DOI: 10.1186/scrt474.

[20] EMA/468680/2018. Public summary of opinion on orphan designation ex-vivo fused autologous human bone marrow-derived mesenchymal stem cell with allogenic human myoblast for the treatment of Duchenne muscular dystrophy. 19 September 2018.

[21] Siemionow M, Szilagyi E, Cwykiel J, Domaszewska-Szostek A, Heydemann A, Garcia-Martinez J, et al. Transplantation of Dystrophin Expressing Chimeric (DEC) Human Cells of Myoblast/MSC Origin Improves Function in Duchenne Muscular Dystrophy Model. Stem Cells Dev 2021; 30(4): 190-202. DOI: 10.1089/scd.2020.0161.

[22] Zhang Y, Miron RJ, Li S, Shi B, Sculean A, Cheng X. Novel MesoPorous BioGlass/silk scaffold containing adPDGF-B and adBMP7 for the repair of periodontal defects in beagle dogs. J Clin Periodontol 2015; 42(3): 262-271. DOI: 10.1111/jcpe.12364.

[23] El-Sayed KMF, Dörfer CE. Animal Models for Periodontal Tissue Engineering: A Knowledge-Generating Process. Tissue Eng Part C Methods 2017; 23(12): 900-925. DOI: 10.1089/ten.TEC.2017.0130.

[24] Bozorgmehr M, Gurung S, Darzi S, Nikoo S, Kazemnejad S, Zarnani AH, et al. Endometrial and Menstrual Blood Mesenchymal Stem/Stromal Cells: Biological Properties and Clinical Application. Front Cell Dev Biol 2020; 8: 497. DOI: 10.3389/fcell.2020.00497.

[25] Kang YH, Lee HJ, Jang SJ, Byun JH, Lee JS, Lee HC, et al. Immunomodulatory properties and in vivo osteogenesis of human dental stem cells from fresh and cryopreserved dental follicles. Differentiation 2015; 90(1-3): 48-58. DOI: 10.1016/j.diff.2015.10.001.

[26] Naji A, Eitoku M, Favier B, Deschaseaux F, Rouas-Freiss N, Suganuma N. Biological functions of mesenchymal stem cells and clinical implications. Cell Mol Life Sci 2019; 76: 3323-3348. DOI: 10.1007/s00018-019-03125-1.

[27] Nikfarjam S, Rezaie J, Zolbanin NM, Jafari R. Mesenchymal stem cell derived-exosomes: a modern approach in translational medicine. J Transl Med 2020; 18: 449. DOI: 10.1186/s12967-020-02622-3.

[28] Jiang W, Xu J. Immune modulation by mesenchymal stem cells. Cell Prolif 2020; 53(1): e12712. DOI: 10.1111/cpr.12712.

[29] Thomas M, Lotfi R, Gjerde C, Mustafa K, Veronesi E, Ahmed AB, et al. Translation of a standardized manufacturing protocol for mesenchymal stromal cells: A systematic comparison of validation and manufacturing data. Cytotherapy 2019; 21: 468-482. DOI: 10.1016/j.jcyt.2019.03.001.

[30] Dominici M, Le Blanc K, Mueller I, Slaper-Cortenbach I, Marini F, Krause D, et al. Minimal criteria for

defining multipotent mesenchymal stromal cells. The International Society for Cellular Therapy position statement. Cytotherapy 2006; 8(4): 315-317. DOI: 10.1080/1465324060 0855905.

[31] Horwitz EM, Le Blanc K, Dominici M, Mueller I, Slaper-Cortenbach I, Marini FC, et al. Clarification of the nomenclature for MSC: The International Society for Cellular Therapy position statement. Cytotherapy 2005; 7(5): 393-395. DOI: 10.1080/14653240500319234.

[32] Pham PV, Vu NB, Pham VM, Truong NH, Pham TLB, Dang LTT, et al. Good manufacturing practice-compliant isolation and culture of human umbilical cord blood-derived mesenchymal stem cells. J Transl Med 2014; 12: 56. DOI: 10.1186/1479-5876-12-56.

[33] Barckhausen C, Rice B, Baila S, Sensebé L, Schrezenmeier H, Nold P, et al. GMP-Compliant Expansion of Clinical-Grade Human Mesenchymal Stromal/Stem Cells Using a Closed Hollow Fiber Bioreactor. Methods Mol Biol 2016; 1416: 389-412. DOI: 10.1007/978-1-4939-3584-0_23.

[34] Tsuchiya S, Chiba M, Kishimoto KN, Nakamura H, Tsuchiya M, Hayashi H. Transfer of the bone morphogenetic protein 4 gene into rat periodontal ligament by in vivo electroporation. Arch Oral Biol 2017; 74: 123-132. DOI: 10.1016/j.archoralbio.2016.11.013.

[35] Park SY, Kim KH, Kim S, Lee YM, Seol YJ. BMP-2 Gene Delivery-Based Bone Regeneration in Dentistry. Pharmaceutics 2019; 11: 393. DOI: 10.3390/pharmaceutics11080393.

[36] Jin Q, Anusaksathien O, Webb SA, Printz MA, Giannobile WV. Engineering of tooth-supporting structures by delivery of PDGF gene therapy vectors. Mol Ther 2004: 9: 519-526. DOI: 10.1016/j.ymthe.2004.01.016.

[37] Tang H, Mattheos N, Yao Y, Jia Y, Ma L, Gong P. In vivo osteoprotegerin gene therapy preventing bone loss induced by periodontitis. J Periodontal Res 2015; 50(4): 434-443. DOI: 10.1111/jre.12224.

[38] Mornet E. Hypophosphatasia. Metabolism 2018; 82: 142-155. DOI: 10.1016/j.metabol.2017.08.013.

[39] Choida V, Bubbear JS. Update on the management of hypophosphatasia. Ther Adv Musculoskel 2019; 11: 1759720X1986399. DOI: 10.1177/1759720X19863997.

[40] Bloch-Zupan A, Vaysse F. Hypophosphatasia: oral cavity and dental disorders. Arch Pédiatrie 2017; 24: 5S80-4. DOI: 10.1016/S0929-693X(18)30020-4.

[41] Bianchi ML, Bishop NJ, Guañabens N, Hofmann, Jakob F, Roux C, et al. Hypophosphatasia in adolescents and adults: overview of diagnosis and treatment. Osteoporos Int 2020; 31(8): 1445-1460. DOI: 10.1007/s00198-020-05345-9.

[42] Stürznickel J, Schmidt FN, Vopelius EV, Delsmann MM, Schmidt C, Jandl NM, et al. Bone healing and reactivation of remodeling under asfotase alfa therapy in adult patients with pediatric-onset hypophosphatasia. Bone 2021; 143: 115794. DOI: 10.1016/j.bone.2020.115794.

[43] Cahill RA, Wenkert D, Perlman SA, Steele A, Coburn SP, McAlister WH, et al. Infantile Hypophosphatasia: Transplantation Therapy Trial Using Bone Fragments and Cultured Osteoblasts. J Clin Endocrinol & Metabolism 2007; 92: 2923-2930. DOI: 10.1210/jc.2006-2131.

[44] Okawa R, Iijima O, Kishino M, Okawa H, Toyosawa S,

Sugano-Tajima H, et al. Gene therapy improves dental manifestations in hypophosphatasia model mice. J Periodontal Res 2017; 52: 471-478. DOI: 10.1111/jre.12412.

[45] Ikeue R, Nakamura-Takahashi A, Nitahara-Kasahara Y, Watanabe A, Muramatsu T, Sato T, et al. Bone-Targeted Alkaline Phosphatase Treatment of Mandibular Bone and Teeth in Lethal Hypophosphatasia via an scAAV8 Vector. Mol Ther-Meth Clin D 2018; 10: 361-370. DOI: 10.1016/j.omtm.2018.08.004.

[46] Nakamura-Takahashi A, Tanase T, Matsunaga S, Shintani S, Abe S, Nitahara-Kasahara Y, et al. High-Level Expression of Alkaline Phosphatase by Adeno-Associated Virus Vector Ameliorates Pathological Bone Structure in a Hypophosphatasia Mouse Model. Calcif Tissue Int 2020; 106(6): 665-677. DOI: 10.1007/s00223-020-00676-5.

[47] Hirashima S, Kanazawa T, Ohta K, Nakamura KI. Three-dimensional ultrastructural imaging and quantitative analysis of the periodontal ligament. Anat Sci Int 2020; 95(1): 1-11. DOI: 10.1007/s12565-019-00502-5.

[48] Li A, Thomas RZ, van der Sluis L, Tjakkes GH, Slot DE. Definitions used for a healthy periodontium-A systematic review. Int J Dent Hyg 2020; 18(4): 327-343. DOI: 10.1111/idh.12438.

[49] Asa'ad F, Monje A, Larsson L. Role of epigenetics in alveolar bone resorption and regeneration around periodontal and peri-implant tissues. Eur J Oral Sci 2019; 127(6): 477-493. DOI: 10.1111/eos.12657.

[50] Zeng WY, Ning Y, Huang X. Advanced technologies in periodontal tissue regeneration based on stem cells: Current status and future perspectives. J Dent Sci 2021; 16(1): 501-507. DOI: 10.1016/j.jds.2020.07.008.

[51] Eggert FM, Levin L. Biology of teeth and implants: Host factors - pathology, regeneration, and the role of stem cells. Quintessence Int 2018; 49(6): 497-509. DOI: 10.3290/j.qi.a40289.

[52] Abukawa H, Terai H, Hannouche D, Vacanti JP, Kaban LB, Troulis MJ. Formation of a mandibular condyle in vitro by tissue engineering. J Oral Maxillofac Surg 2003; 61(1): 94-100. DOI: 10.1053/joms.2003.50015.

[53] Abukawa H, Shin M, Williams WB, Vacanti JP, Kaban LB, Troulis MJ. Reconstruction of Mandibular Defects with Autologous Tissue-Engineered Bone. J Oral Maxillofac Surg 2004; 62: 601-606. DOI: 10.1016/j.joms.2003.11.010.

[54] Streckbein P, Jäckel S, Malik CY, Obert M, Kähling C, Wilbrand JF, et al. Reconstruction of critical-size mandibular defects in immunoin competent rats with human adipose-derived stromal cells. J Oral Maxillofac Surg 2013; 41(6): 496-503. DOI: 10.1016/j.jcms.2013.04.002.

[55] Compston JE, McClung MR, Leslie WD. Osteoporosis. Lancet 2019; 393(10169): 364-376. DOI: 10.1016/S0140-6736(18)32112-3.

[56] Cheng C, Wentworth K, Shoback DM. New Frontiers in Osteoporosis Therapy. Annu Rev Med 2020; 71(1): 277-288. DOI: 10.1146/annurev-med-052218-020620.

[57] Arjmand B, Sarvari M, Alavi-Moghadam S, Payab M, Goodarzi P, Gilany K, et al. Prospect of Stem Cell Therapy and Regenerative Medicine in Osteoporosis. Front Endocrinol 2020; 11: 430. DOI: 10.3389/fendo.2020.00430.

[58] Huijuan Liu, Xuechun Xia, Baojie Li. Mesenchymal stem cell aging: Mechanisms and influences on skeletal and non-skeletal tissues. Exp Biol Med

(Maywood) 2015; 240(8): 1099-1106. DOI: 10.1177/1535370215591828.

[59] Li D, Zhou W, Cao M. Periostin-modified bone marrow mesenchymal stem cells from osteoporotic rats promote alveolar bone regeneration. J Mol Histol 2019; 50: 493-502. DOI: 10.1007/s10735-019-09843-x.

[60] Sui B, Hu C, Zhang X, Zhao P, He T, Zhou C, et al. Allogeneic Mesenchymal Stem Cell Therapy Promotes Osteoblastogenesis and Prevents Glucocorticoid-Induced Osteoporosis. Stem Cells Transl Med 2016; 5(9): 1238-1246. DOI: 10.5966/sctm.2015-0347.

[61] Kiernan J, Hu S, Grynpas MD, Davies JE, Stanford WL. Systemic Mesenchymal Stromal Cell Transplantation Prevents Functional Bone Loss in a Mouse Model of Age-Related Osteoporosis: MSC Transplantation Prevents Bone Loss. Stem Cells Transl Med 2016; 5(5): 683-693. DOI: 10.5966/sctm.2015-0231.

[62] Xu R, Fu Z, Liu X, Xiao T, Zhang P, Du Y, et al. Transplantation of osteoporotic bone marrow stromal cells rejuvenated by the overexpression of SATB2 prevents alveolar bone loss in ovariectomized rats. Exp Gerontol 2016; 84: 71-79. DOI: 10.1016/j.exger.2016.09.001.

[63] Chang J, Hakam AE, McCauley LK. Current Understanding of the Pathophysiology of Osteonecrosis of the Jaw. Curr Osteoporos Rep 2018; 16(5): 584-595. DOI: 10.1007/s11914-018-0474-4.

[64] Anesi A, Generali L, Sandoni L, Pozzi S, Alexis Grande A. From Osteoclast Differentiation to Osteonecrosis of the Jaw: Molecular and Clinical Insights. Int J Mol Sci 2019; 20(19): 4925. DOI: 10.3390/ijms20194925.

[65] He L, Sun X, Liu Z, Qiu Y, Niu Y. Pathogenesis and multidisciplinary management of medication-related osteonecrosis of the jaw. Int J Oral Sci 2020; 12(1): 30. DOI: 10.1038/s41368-020-00093-2.

[66] Melguizo-Rodríguez L, Costela-Ruiz VJ, Manzano-Moreno FJ, Ruiz C, Illescas-Montes R. Salivary Biomarkers and Their Application in the Diagnosis and Monitoring of the Most Common Oral Pathologies. Int J Mol Sci 2020; 21(14): 5173. DOI: 10.3390/ijms21145173.

[67] Vannala V, Palaian S, Shankar PR. Therapeutic Dimensions of Bisphosphonates: A Clinical Update. Int J Prev Med 2020; 11: 166. DOI: 10.4103/ijpvm.IJPVM_33_19.

[68] Srivastava A, Nogueras-Gonzalez GM, Geng Y, Won AM, Cabanillas ME, Naing A, et al. Prevalence of medication related osteonecrosis of the jaw in patients treated with sequential antiresorptive drugs: systematic review and meta-analysis. Support Care Cancer 2020. DOI: 10.1007/s00520-020-05882-3.

[69] Endo Y, Funayama H, Yamaguchi K, Monma Y, Yu Z, Deng X, et al. Basic Studies on the Mechanism, Prevention, and Treatment of Osteonecrosis of the Jaw Induced by Bisphosphonates. Yakugaku Zasshi 2020; 140(1): 63-79. DOI: 10.1248/yakushi.19-00125.

[70] Steel BJ. Management of Medication-related Osteonecrosis of the Jaw (MRONJ) risk in patients due to commence anti-resorptive/anti-angiogenic drugs - how should pre-drug-treatment dental preventive care be organised?. Community Dent Health 2019; 36(4): 244-254. DOI: 10.1922/CDH_4582Steel11.

[71] Wan JT, Sheeley DM, Somerman MJ, Lee JS. Mitigating osteonecrosis of the jaw (ONJ) through preventive dental

care and understanding of risk factors. Bone Res 2020; 8: 14. DOI: 10.1038/s41413-020-0088-1.

[72] d'Aquino, R., De Rosa, A., Lanza, V., Tirino, V., Laino, L., Graziano, A., et al. Human mandible bone defect repair by the grafting of dental pulp stem/progenitor cells and collagen sponge biocomplexes. Eur Cell Mater 2009; 18(7): 75-83. DOI: 10.22203/ecm.v018a07.

[73] Li, Y., Xu, J., Mao, L., Liu, Y., Gao, R., Zheng, Z., et al. Allogeneic mesenchymal stem cell therapy for bisphosphonate-related jaw osteonecrosis in swine. Stem Cells Dev 2013; 22(14): 2047-2056. DOI: 10.1089/scd.2012.0615.

[74] Barba-Recreo P, Del Castillo-Pardo JL, Georgiev-Hristov T, Bravo-Burguillos ER, Abarrategi A, Burgueño M, et al. Adipose-derived stem cells and platelet-rich plasma for preventive treatment of bisphosphonate-related osteonecrosis of the jaw in a murine model. J Craniomaxillofac Surg 2015; 43(7): 1161-1168. DOI: 10.1016/j.jcms.2015.04.026.

[75] Alonso-Rodriguez E, González-Martín-Moro J, Cebrián-Carretero JL, Del Castillo-Pardo L, Pozo-Kreilinger JJ, Ruiz-Bravo E, et al. Bisphosphonate-related osteonecrosis. Application of adipose-derived stem cells in an experimental murine model. Med Oral Patol Oral Cir Bucal 2019; 24(4): e529–e536. DOI: 10.4317/medoral.22959.

[76] U.S. National Library of Medicine. Use of Autologous Bone Marrow Stem Cells Seeded on Porous Tricalcium Phosphate Matrix and Demineralized Bone Matrix in Patients with Osteonecrosis (MSC/ONM). ClinicalTrials.gov *identifier:* NCT02566681. Available from: https://www.clinicaltrials.gov/ct2/show/NCT02566681?term=NCT02566681&draw=2&rank=1

[77] Herdman M, Badia X, Berra S. EuroQol-5D: a simple alternative for measuring health-related quality of life in primary care. Aten Primaria 2001; 28(6): 425-430. DOI: 10.1016/s0212-6567(01)70406-4.

[78] Farzadmoghadam M, Mohammadi TM, Goudarzi R, Mohammadi M, Hasheminejad N. Is there a relationship between general and oral health-related quality of life in partially edentulous patients before and after implant treatment? A quasi-experimental study. Clin Oral Implants Res 2020; 31(6): 557-564. DOI: 10.1111/clr.13593.

[79] Gundestrup AK, Lynggaard CD, Forner L, Heino TJ, Jakobsen KK, Fischer-Nielsen A, et al. Mesenchymal Stem Cell Therapy for Osteo radionecrosis of the Mandible: a Systematic Review of Preclinical and Human Studies. Stem Cell Reviews and Reports 2020; 16: 1208-1221. DOI: 10.1007/s12015-020-10034-5.

[80] Matsuo A, Chiba H, Takahashi H, Toyoda J, Hasegawa O, Hojo S. Bone quality of mandibles reconstructed with particulate cellular bone and marrow, and platelet-rich plasma. J Craniomaxillofac Surg 2011; 39(8): 628-632. DOI: 10.1016/j.jcms.2011.01.003.

[81] Trautvetter W, Kaps C, Schmelzeisen R, Sauerbier S, Sittinger M. Tissue-engineered polymer-based periosteal bone grafts for maxillary sinus augmentation: five-year clinical results. J Oral Maxillofac Surg 2011; 69: 2753-2762. DOI: 10.1016/j.joms.2011.02.096.

[82] Matichescu A, Ardelean LC, Rusu LC, Craciun D, Bratu EA, Babucea M, et al. Advanced Biomaterials and Techniques for Oral Tissue

Engineering and Regeneration-A Review. Materials (Basel) 2020; 13(22): 5303. DOI: 10.3390/ma13225303.

[83] Zheng C, Chen J, Liu S, Jin Y. Stem cell-based bone and dental regeneration: a view of microenvironmental modulation. Int J Oral Sci 2019; 11(3): 23. DOI: 10.1038/s41368-019-0060-3.

[84] Sui BD, Zheng CX, Li M, Jin Y, Hu CH. Epigenetic Regulation of Mesenchymal Stem Cell Homeostasis. Trends Cell Biol 2020; 30(2): 97-116. DOI: 10.1016/j.tcb.2019.11.006.

[85] Khayambashi P, Iyer J, Pillai S, Upadhyay A, Zhang Y, Tran SD. Hydrogel Encapsulation of Mesenchymal Stem Cells and Their Derived Exosomes for Tissue Engineering. Int J Mol Sci 2021; 22(2): E684. DOI: 10.3390/ijms22020684.

[86] Lee JWY, Bance ML. Physiology of Osseointegration. Otolaryngol Clin North Am 2019; 52(2): 231-242. DOI: 10.1016/j.otc.2018.11.004.

[87] Weng CC, Ou KL, Wu CY, Huang YH, Wang J, Yen Y, et al. Mechanism and Clinical Properties of StemBios Cell Therapy: Induction of Early Osseointegration in Novel Dental Implants. Int J Oral Maxillofac Implants 2017; 32(1): e47-e54. DOI: 10.11607/jomi.4460.

[88] Alqahtani NA, Chandra moorthy HC, Shaik S, Syed J, Chowdhary R, Antony L. Bone Marrow Mesenchymal Stromal Cells (BMMSCs) Augment Osteointegration of Dental Implants in Type 1 Diabetic Rabbits: An X-Ray Micro-Computed Tomographic Evaluation. Medicina (Kaunas) 2020; 56(4): 148. DOI: 10.3390/medicina56040148.

[89] Gan L, Liu Y, Cui D, Pan Y, Zheng L, Wan M. Dental Tissue-Derived Human Mesenchymal Stem Cells and Their Potential in Therapeutic Application. Stem Cells Int 2020; 1-17. DOI: 10.1155/2020/8864572.

[90] Xiao Z, Lei T, Liu Y, Yang Y, Bi W, Du H. The potential therapy with dental tissue-derived mesenchymal stem cells in Parkinson's disease. Stem Cell Res Ther 2021; 12(1): 5. DOI: 10.1186/s13287-020-01957-4.

[91] Shanbhag S, Suliman S, Pandis N, Stavropoulos A, Sanz M, Mustafa K. Cell therapy for orofacial bone regeneration: A systematic review and meta-analysis. J Clin Periodontol 2019; 46: 162-182. DOI: 10.1111/jcpe.13049.

[92] Vidal B, Pinto A, Galvão MJ, Santos AR, Rodrigues A, Cascão R, et al. Bone histomorphometry revisited. Acta Reumatol Port 2012; 37(4): 294-300. PMID: 24126421.

[93] Mehta S, Blagg R, Willcockson J, Gociman B, Yamashiro D, Siddiqi F. Cost-effectiveness analysis of demineralized bone matrix and rhBMP-2 versus autologous iliac crest bone grafting in alveolar cleft patients. Plast Reconstr Surg 2018; 142: 737-743. DOI: 10.1097/PRS.0000000000004646.

[94] Gjerde C, Mustafa K, Hellem S, Rojewski M, Gjengedal H, Yassin MA, et al. Cell therapy induced regeneration of severely atrophied mandibular bone in a clinical trial. Stem Cell Res Ther 2018; 9(1): 213. DOI: 10.1186/s13287-018-0951-9.

[95] U.S. National Library of Medicine. Reconstruction of Jaw Bone Using Mesenchymal Stem Cells. ClinicalTrials.gov *identifier:* NCT02751125. Available from: https://www.clinicaltrials.gov/ct2/show/NCT02751125?term=NCT02751125&draw=2&rank=1

[96] Al-Jetaily S, Al-Dosari AA. Assessment of Osstell™ and Periotest® systems in measuring dental implant stability (in vitro study). Saudi Dent J

2011; 23(1): 17-21. DOI: 10.1016/j.sdentj.2010.09.003.

[97] U.S. National Library of Medicine. Efficacy in Alveolar Bone Regeneration With Autologous MSCs and Biomaterial in Comparison to Autologous Bone Grafting (Maxibone). ClinicalTrials.gov *identifier:* NCT04297813. Available from: https://www.clinicaltrials.gov/ct2/show/NCT04297813?term=NCT04297813&draw=2&rank=1

[98] Karcioglu O, Topacoglu H, Dikme O, Dikme O. A systematic review of the pain scales in adults: Which to use? Am J Emerg Med 2018; 36: 707-714. DOI: 10.1016/j.ajem.2018.01.008.

[99] Jacobs R, Salmon B, Codari M, Hassan B, Bornstein MM. Cone beam computed tomography in implant dentistry: recommendations for clinical use. BMC Oral Health 2018; 18: 88. DOI: 10.1186/s12903-018-0523-5.

[100] Liras A. Biological therapies for inherited diseases: social and bioethical considerations. Hemophilia as an example. Expert Opin Biol Ther 2015; 15: 713-722. DOI: 10.1517/14712598.2015.1029451.

[101] Staples RJ, Ivanovski S, Cedryck Vaquette. Fibre guiding scaffolds for periodontal tissue engineering. J Periodontal Res 2020; 55(3): 331-341. DOI: 10.1111/jre.12729.

[102] Liras A. Future research and therapeutic applications of human stem cells: general, regulatory, and bioethical aspects. J Transl Med 2010; 8: 131. DOI: 10.1186/1479-5876-8-131.

[103] Petrini C. Bioethics of Clinical Applications of Stem Cells. Int J Mol Sci 2017; 18: 814. DOI: 10.3390/ijms18040814.

[104] Bakopoulou A. Prospects of Advanced Therapy Medicinal Products-Based Therapies in Regenerative Dentistry: Current Status, Comparison with Global Trends in Medicine, and Future Perspectives. J Endod 2020; 46: S175-SS88. DOI: 10.1016/j.joen.2020.06.026.

[105] Watt RG, Daly B, Allison P, Macpherson LMD, Venturelli R, Listl S, et al. Ending the neglect of global oral health: time for radical action. Lancet 2019; 394: 261-272. DOI: 10.1016/S0140-6736(19)31133-X.

[106] Peres MA, Macpherson LMD, Weyant RJ, Daly B, Venturelli R, Mathur MR, et al. Oral diseases: a global public health challenge. Lancet 2019; 394: 249-260. DOI: 10.1016/S0140-6736(19)31146-8.

[107] Joshi C, Bapat R, Anderson W, Dawson D, Hijazi K, Cherukara G. Detection of periodontal microorganisms in coronary atheromatous plaque specimens of myocardial infarction patients: a systematic review and metanalysis. Trends Cardiovasc Med 2021; 31: 69-82. DOI: 10.1016/j.tcm.2019.12.005.

[108] Srivastava MC, Srivastava R, Verma PK, Gautam A. Metabolic syndrome and periodontal disease: an overview for physicians. J Family Med Prim Care 2019; 8: 3492-3495. DOI: 10.4103/jfmpc.jfmpc_866_19.

[109] Bagegni A, Abou-Ayash S, Rücker G, Algarny A, Att W. The influence of prosthetic material on implant and prosthetic survival of implant-supported fixed complete dentures: a systematic review and metanalysis. J Prosthodont Res 2019; 63: 251-265. DOI: 10.1016/j.jpor.2019.02.001.

[110] Shi X, Mao J, Liu Y. Pulp stem cells derived from human permanent and deciduous teeth: biological characteristics and therapeutic applications. Stem Cells Transl Med 2020; 9: 445-464. DOI: 10.1002/sctm.19-0398.

[111] Eder C, Wild C. Technology forecast: advanced therapies in late clinical research, EMA approval or clinical application via hospital exemption. J Mark Access Health Policy 2019; 7: 1600939. DOI: 10.1080/20016689.2019.1600939.

[112] Boráň T, Menezes-Ferreira M, Reischl I, Celis P, Ferry N, Gänsbacher B, et al. Clinical development and commercialization of advanced therapy medicinal products in the European Union: how are the product pipeline and regulatory framework evolving? Hum Gene Ther Clin Dev 2017; 28: 126-135. DOI: 10.1089/humc.2016.193.

[113] Pieri AD, Ribeiro S, Tsiapalis D, Eglin D, Bohner M, Dubruel P, et al. Joint academic and industrial efforts towards innovative and efficient solutions for clinical needs. J Mater Sci Mater Med 2018; 29: 129. DOI: 10.1007/s10856-018-6136-3.

[114] Regulation (EC) No. 1394/2007 of the European Parliament and of the Council on Advanced Therapy Medicinal Products and amending Directive 2001/83/EC and Regulation (EC) No. 726/ 2004. OJ L 2007; 324: 121-137.

[115] Directive 2009/120/EC amending Directive 2001/83/EC of the European Parliament and of the Council on the Community code relating to medicinal products for human use as regards advanced therapy medicinal products. OJ L 2009; 242: 3-12.

[116] Therapeutic goods administration, Australia's regulatory framework for biological. [cited April 05, 2021]. Available from: http://www.tga.gov.au/industry/biologicals-framework.htm.

[117] Health Canada's guidance document for cell, tissue and organ establishments safety of human cells, tissues and organs for transplantation. [cited April 05, 2021]. Available from: http://www.hc-sc.gc.ca/dhp-mps/brgtherap/reg-init/cell/cto_gd_ld-eng.php.

[118] FDA's cellular therapy guidance documents. [cited April 05, 2021]. Available from: http://www.fda.gov/BiologicsBlood.

[119] Korea's Ministry of Food and Drug Safety, Cell and Gene Therapy Products division. Regulation of Cell and Gene Therapy Products in Korea. [cited April 05, 2021]. Available from: https://www.mfds.go.kr/eng/wpge/m_22/de011012l001.do.

[120] Singapore's Ministry of Health, Health Sciences Authority. Guidance on therapeutic product registration in Singapore [cited April 05, 2021]. Available from: https://www.hsa.gov.sg/content/hsa/en/Health_Products_Regulation/Western_Medicines/Overview/Guidelines_on_Drug_Registration.html.

[121] Japan Pharmaceutical Manufacturers Association, Regulatory Information Task Force. Pharmaceutical Administration and Regulations in Japan: Information on Japanese Regulatory Affairs. [cited April 05, 2021]. Available from: Japan: http://www.jpma.or.jp/english/parj/pdf/2019.pdf.

[122] Chisholm J, Crystal C, Viswanathan S. Current state of Health Canada regulation for cellular and gene therapy products: potential cures on the horizon. Cytotherapy 2019; 21(7): 686-698. DOI: 10.1016/j.jcyt.2019.03.005.

[123] Directive 2003/94/EC laying down the principles and guidelines of good manufacturing practice in respect of medicinal products for human use and investigational medicinal products for human use. OJ L 2003; 262: 22-26.

[124] Caplan AI, Mason C, Reeve B. The 3Rs of cell therapy. Stem Cells Transl Med 2017; 6: 17-21. DOI: 10.5966/sctm.2016-0180.

[125] Corbett MS, Webster A, Hawkins R, Woolacott N. Innovative regenerative medicines in the EU: a better future in evidence? BMC Med 2017; 15: 49. DOI: 10.1186/s12916-017-0818-4.